Pain, Analgesia and Anesthesia

Guest Editor

VALERIE GIRARD-POWELL, RN

PERIOPERATIVE NURSING CLINICS

www.periopnursing.theclinics.com

Consulting Editor
NANCY GIRARD, PhD, RN, FAAN

December 2009 • Volume 4 • Number 4

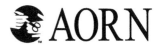

SAUNDERS an imprint of ELSEVIER, Inc.

W.B. SAUNDERS COMPANY

A Division of Elsevier Inc.

1600 John F. Kennedy Boulevard • Suite 1800 • Philadelphia, Pennsylvania 19103-2899

http://www.periopnursing.theclinics.com

PERIOPERATIVE NURSING CLINICS Volume 4, Number 4
December 2009 ISSN 1556-7931, ISBN-13: 978-1-4377-1749-5

Editor: Katie Hartner
Developmental Editor: Donald Mumford

Perioperative Nursing Clinics (ISSN 1556-7931) is published quarterly by Elsevier, 360 Park Avenue South, New York, NY 10010. Months of issue are March, June, September and December. Business and Editorial Offices: 1600 John F. Kennedy Blvd., Suite 1800, Philadelphia, PA 19103-2899. Customer Service Office: 11830 Westline Industrial Drive, St. Louis, MO 63146. Periodicals postage paid at New York, NY and at additional mailing offices. Subscription prices are $116.00 per year (domestic individuals), $213.00 per year (domestic institutions), $58.00 per year (domestic students/residents), $150 per year (international individuals), $245 per year (international institutions), and $62.00 per year (International students/residents). Foreign air speed delivery is included in all *Clinics* subscription prices. All prices are subject to change without notice. **POSTMASTER:** Send change of address to *Perioperative Nursing Clinics*, Customer Service (orders, claims, online, change of address): Elsevier Periodicals Customer Service, 11830 Westline Industrial Drive, St. Louis, MO 63146. Tel: 1-800-654-2452 (U.S. and Canada). Fax: 314-523-5170. E-mail: journalscustomer service-usa@elsevier.com (for print support); journalsonlinesupport-usa@elsevier.com (for online support).

Reprints. For copies of 100 or more, of articles in this publication, please contact the Commercial Rights Department, Elsevier Inc., 360 Park Avenue South, New York, NY 10010-1710; phone: (+1) 212-633-3813; fax: (+1) 212-462-1935; e-mail: reprints@elsevier.com.

Printed and bound by CPI Group (UK) Ltd, Croydon, CR0 4YY

Transferred to Digital Print 2011

Contributors

GUEST EDITOR

VALERIE GIRARD-POWELL, RN
Perioperative Registered Nurse, Liver Transplant Clinical Coordinator, Operating Room RN, University Transplant Center, San Antonio, Texas

AUTHORS

STACY ACKERLIND, PhD
Student Affairs, University of Utah, Salt Lake City, Utah

ANKITA AGARWAL, BS
Translational Pain Research and Neuromedicine Pain Management Center, Department of Neurosurgery, University of Rochester School of Medicine and Dentistry, Rochester, New York

RICHARD A. BAUM, MD
Division of Angiography and Interventional Radiology, Department of Radiology, Brigham and Women's Hospital, Harvard Medical School, Boston, Massachusetts

RINIA L. CRUZ, CRNA
Anesthesia Specialist, Department of Anesthesiology, University of Texas Health Science Center at San Antonio, San Antonio, Texas

WILLEM J.S. DE VILLIERS, MD, PhD, MHCM
Division of Digestive Diseases and Nutrition, Department of Internal Medicine, University of Kentucky Medical Center, University of Kentucky College of Medicine, Lexington, Kentucky

NASR ENANY, MD
Department of Anesthesiology, University of Cincinnati College of Medicine, Cincinnati, Ohio

REGINA Y. FRAGNETO, MD
Professor, Department of Anesthesiology, University of Kentucky College of Medicine, Lexington, Kentucky

SAMUEL M. GALVAGNO, DO
Critical Care Fellow, Johns Hopkins University School of Medicine, Baltimore, Maryland

DANIEL T. GOULSON, MD
Professor; Director of Ambulatory Anesthesia, Department of Anesthesiology, University of Kentucky College of Medicine, Lexington, Kentucky

ROSS HANSON, BS
Research Fellow, Translational Pain Research and Neuromedicine Pain Management Center, Department of Neurosurgery, University of Rochester School of Medicine and Dentistry, Rochester, New York

STEVEN H. HOROWITZ, MD
The University of Vermont College of Medicine, Burlington, Vermont; Department
of Neurology, Massachusetts General Hospital, Boston, Massachusetts

NANCY M. KANE, DBA
Professor of Management, Harvard School of Public Health, Boston, Massachusetts

KENNETH L. KIRSH, PhD
Pharmacy Practice and Science, University of Kentucky, Lexington, Kentucky

BHAVANI-SHANKAR KODALI, MD
Associate Professor, Harvard Medical School; Clinical Director, Department
of Anesthesiology and Perioperative, and Pain Medicine, Brigham and Woman's Hospital,
Boston, Massachusetts

ELIZABETH DEMERS LAVELLE, MD
Assistant Professor, Department of Anesthesia, SUNY Upstate Medical University,
Syracuse, New York

WILLIAM F. LAVELLE, MD
Assistant Professor, Department of Orthopaedics, SUNY Upstate Medical University,
Syracuse, New York

JOHN D. MARKMAN, MD
Associate Professor of Neurosurgery, Director, Translational Pain Research and
Neuromedicine Pain Management Center, Department of Neurosurgery,
University of Rochester School of Medicine and Dentistry, Rochester, New York

RAMON MARTIN, MD
Department of Anesthesiology, Perioperative and Pain Medicine, Brigham and Women's
Hospital, Harvard Medical School, Boston, Massachusetts

GARY McCLEANE, MD
Rampark Pain Centre, Hurgan, Northern Ireland, United Kingdom

TANIA V. MEHTA, CRNA
Anesthesia Specialist, Department of Anesthesiology, University of Texas Health Science
Center at San Antonio, San Antonio, Texas

MUHAMMAD A. MUNIR, MD
Department of Anesthesiology, University of Cincinnati College of Medicine, Cincinnati,
Ohio

AKIKO OKIFUJI, PhD
Professor, Pain Research and Management Center, Department of Anesthesiology,
University of Utah, Salt Lake City, Utah

ANNIE PHILIP, MD
Department of Anesthesiology, University of Rochester School of Medicine and Dentistry,
Rochester, New York

MATTHEW P. SCHENKER, MD
Division of Angiography and Interventional Radiology, Department of Radiology, Brigham
and Women's Hospital, Harvard Medical School, Boston, Massachusetts

PAUL B. SHYN, MD
Division of Abdominal Imaging and Intervention, Department of Radiology, Brigham and Women's Hospital, Harvard Medical School, Boston, Massachusetts

HOWARD S. SMITH, MD, FACP
Department of Anesthesiology, Albany Medical College, Albany, New York

JUN-MING ZHANG, MSc, MD
Department of Anesthesiology, University of Cincinnati College of Medicine, Cincinnati, Ohio

Contents

Pain is a complex, idiosyncratic experience. When pain is the primary complaint for seeking medical attention, understanding of multiple factors is essential in guiding successful treatment. Behavioral medicine, a branch of psychology, has been an integral part of interdisciplinary/multidisciplinay care of pain patients. In this article, we provide an overview of behavioral medicine approaches to pain, including assessment and commonly used therapeutic methods. Particular attention is given to cognitive-behavioral therapy and motivational enhancement therapy.

Neuropathic pain is initiated or caused by damage or dysfunction of the peripheral or central nervous systems in various disorders, each having pain-related symptoms and signs thought secondary to common pain mechanisms. Ancillary testing may demonstrate associated nervous system abnormalities, however its specificity is inadequate at present, as it makes inferential conclusions from indirect data. Symptom assessment and physical findings remain paramount in the diagnosis of neuropathic pain.

This article reviews the evidence for several common procedural techniques for the treatment of chronic pain, including intraspinal delivery of analgesics, reversible blockade with local anesthetics, augmentation with spinal cord and motor cortex stimulation, and ablation with radiofrequency energy or neurolytic agents. The role of these techniques is defined within the framework of a multidisciplinary approach to the neurobehavioral syndrome of chronic pain. Challenges to the study of the analgesic efficacy of procedural interventions are explored, as are the practical issues raised by their clinical implementation with the aim of helping nonspecialist physicians identify the patients most likely to benefit from these approaches.

Painful conditions of the musculoskeletal system, including myofascial pain syndrome, constitute some of the most important chronic problems encountered in a clinical practice. A myofascial trigger point is a hyperirritable spot, usually within a taut band of skeletal muscle, which is painful on compression and can give rise to characteristic referred pain, motor dysfunction, and autonomic phenomena. Trigger points may be relieved through noninvasive measures, such as spray and stretch, transcutaneous electrical stimulation, physical therapy, and massage. Invasive treatments for myofascial trigger points include injections with local anesthetics, corticosteroids, or botulism toxin or dry needling. The etiology, pathophysiology, and treatment of myofascial trigger points are addressed in this article.

The field of pain medicine is experiencing increased pressure from regulatory agencies and other sources regarding the continuation, or even initial use, of opioids in pain patients. Therefore, it is essential that pain clinicians provide rationale for engaging in this modality of treatment and provide ample documentation in this regard. Thus, assessment and documentation are cornerstones for both protecting your practice and obtaining optimal patient outcomes while on opioid therapy. Several potential tools and documentation strategies are discussed that will aid clinicians in providing evidence for the continuation of this type of treatment for their patients.

Nonopioid analgesics represent a varied collection of analgesic agents, many of which also possess antipyretic or anti-inflammatory actions. As a group, nonopioid analgesics represent reasonable first-line analgesics for a variety of mild to moderate painful conditions and also often may be useful in conjunction with other analgesics (eg, opioids) for a myriad of severe painful conditions. Clinicians treating pain should be familiar with the actions, adverse effects, and individual agents in the group of nonopioid analgesics.

Historically, analgesics were applied by the topical route of administration. With the advent of oral formulations of drugs, topical application became less popular among physicians, although patients still rated this method of drug delivery as efficacious and practical. We now appreciate that peripheral mechanisms of actions of a variety of preparations rationalizes their topical application and gives further opportunity to target peripheral

receptors and neural pathways that previously required systemic administration to achieve therapeutic effect. Therefore, a peripheral effect can be
generated by using locally applied drug and, consequently, systemic concentrations of that drug may not reach the level at which systemic side effects can occur.

practice of modern medicine. The growth and diversity of these non-OR procedures presents unique challenges and opportunities to anesthesiologists and interventional radiologists alike. Collaborative action has led to better patient care and quality management. This discussion considers some angiographic and cross-sectional IR procedures in more detail and comments on some of the anesthesia choices and considerations. In addition, specific concerns regarding anesthesia in the area of IR are reviewed.

Nancy M. Kane

Achieving fundamental reform of the health care system to improve patient outcomes will take decades of effort and a major shift in financial, medical, and political behaviors that have built up since the beginning of health insurance in the United States. To the extent that the present payment systems contribute to the high cost, poor quality, and lack of accountability that characterizes today's health care delivery system, there is hope that reforms are within reach.

THE CLINICS ARE NOW AVAILABLE ONLINE!

Access your subscription at:
www.theclinics.com

Preface

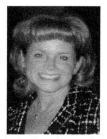

Valerie Girard-Powell, RN
Guest Editor

Recent advances in medicine and technology have led to a shift from surgical procedures that demand hospital operating room time to those performed in outpatient settings, office clinics, and day surgical centers. The shift allows physicians and patients greater flexibility, faster procedural times, and shorter sedation times and often incurs less expense for physicians and patients. Although convenient for patients and physicians, new challenges that must be considered to maintain patient satisfaction and safety are posed in light of these changes.

One major change is the shift from anesthesiologists or certified registered nurse (RN) anesthetists to a RN providing sedation or conscious sedation for these patients. Some settings may have an anesthetic care provider available in the building in the event of a circumstance that requires emergent care of a formally trained anesthetic care provider. Other institutions employ a RN who works under the supervision of the physician performing the procedure to provide sedation.

RNs without advanced training in sedation and airway management can quickly become overwhelmed in an unforeseen circumstance, posing a threat to patients and RNs. One example is when too much sedation is inadvertently given, causing a patient to lose the ability to maintain a patent airway. This can lead to a great risk in patient safety. Surgical care providers must strive to maintain the same standards of care for these patients as those that are mandated for them in the operating room setting. RNs performing monitoring and sedation in nonhospital settings must have advanced training, knowledge, and skill sets to properly provide safe and efficient pain relief during the procedures and to achieve optimum levels of sedation needed while preventing critical incidents perioperatively. The practice should include the best possible patient monitoring equipment and RNs must be properly educated or certified, ensuring their ability to quickly identify patients in distress and have a plan of care readily available in the event of an emergency.

RNs are allotted a level of autonomy practicing within the prepared scope of practice under their license. This demands constant reassessment of individual skills and knowledge base as practice settings change. Ways to facilitate exceptional care include remaining current in the latest techniques, advances, and knowledge and always serving as the greatest advocate for patient safety and well being, voicing concerns if they feel patient safety is compromised. All care providers should strive to work toward the goal of encouraging communication and collaboration between

Perioperative Nursing Clinics 4 (2009) xiii–xiv
doi:10.1016/j.cpen.2009.09.012
1556-7931/09/$ – see front matter © 2009 Elsevier Inc. All rights reserved.
periopnursing.theclinics.com

staff and physicians with whom they work during these procedures and implement procedure protocols and uniform standard of care practices in accordance with guidelines from the American Society of Anesthesiologists, the Association of PeriOperative Registered Nurses, and the American Association of Nurse Anesthetists. Nurses must demand advanced training and continued education to provide the excellence in nursing that patients deserve.

This issue of *Perioperative Nursing Clinics* provides various outlooks on the situations encountered with pain control and sedation as surgical procedures move out of the traditional operating room. Certified registered nurse anesthetists provide opinion and recommendations to better prepare these nurses. Well-qualified staff enable facilities to provide excellent patient care while maintaining safe sedation, recovery, and optimum pain management. I hope you enjoy this excellent collection of articles compiled in this issue and apply ideas and suggestions put forth to advance your nursing practice and patient care.

Valerie Girard-Powell, RN
University Transplant Center
4502 Medical Drive MS 18
San Antonio, TX 78229, USA

E-mail address:
valerie.girard@uhs-sa.com

Commentary: Do No Harm

Recent technologic advances in anesthesia have facilitated moving procedures on complex patients, previously performed only in an operating room, to outside an operating room (OOR). The physiologic monitoring standards for these intricate procedures, however, have not evolved concomitantly. Galvagno and Kodali[1] note that studies have suggested that adverse events occurring during procedures performed OOR have a higher severity of injury and may result from lack of adherence to minimum monitoring guidelines. To achieve optimal outcomes in operational efficiency, clinical competence, and patient safety, effective preprocedural evaluation and preparation are critical. Bader and Pothier[2] recommend three key areas of preprocedural preparation for anesthetists working in OORs: (1) a thorough understanding of the techniques and goals of the procedure, (2) familiarity with the arrangement of anesthetizing location, and (3) appropriate prescreening of the patients by an anesthetic provider. Any anesthesia provider not familiar with these preparation techniques will be at a disadvantage and not be able to optimize the anesthetic care for a procedure. In situations where a provider is not specialty trained in sedation and anesthesia, that individual is at a greater disadvantage due to the lack of knowledge regarding pharmacodynamics, pharmokinectics, and airway skills. Besides unfamiliarity with preprocedural preparation, that individual will not have the knowledge base to appropriately handle complex drug interactions, hemodynamic fluctuations, and, most importantly, airway compromise. To ensure a safe environment for providers and patients, there is a need to (1) implement monitoring standards for all procedures performed OOR and to bring them into alignment with those of the operating room, (2) standardize specialty training for providers (not certified registered nurse anesthetist or anesthesiologists) who provide sedation and anesthesia OOR, and (3) maintain a continuing education program for these providers to ensure clinical competence.

Rinia L. Cruz, CRNA
Anesthesia Specialist
Department of Anesthesiology
University of Texas Health Science Center at San Antonio
7703 Floyd Curl Drive
San Antonio, TX 78229

Tania V. Mehta, CRNA
Anesthesia Specialist
Department of Anesthesiology
University of Texas Health Science Center at San Antonio
7703 Floyd Curl Drive
San Antonio, TX 78229

E-mail addresses:
cruzr2@uthscsa.edu (R.L. Cruz)
mehtat@uthscsa.edu (T.V. Mehta)

Perioperative Nursing Clinics 4 (2009) xv–xvi
doi:10.1016/j.cpen.2009.09.013
1556-7931/09/$ – see front matter © 2009 Elsevier Inc. All rights reserved.

REFERENCES

1. Galvagno SM, Kodali K. Critical monitoring issues outside the operating room. Anesthesiol Clin 2009;27:141–56.
2. Bader AM, Pothier NM. Critical monitoring issues outside the operating room. Anesthesiol Clin 2009;27:121–6.

Behavioral Approaches to Pain Management

Akiko Okifuji, PhD[a],*, Stacy Ackerlind, PhD[b]

KEYWORDS

• Behavioral medicine • Psychology • Pain

In the early 1970s, the term "behavioral medicine" began appearing in the literature as a branch of behavioral science that applies scientific knowledge and techniques to prevention, diagnosis, treatment, and rehabilitation of physical illness and maintenance of physical health.[1] A fundamental aspect of behavioral medicine is the recognition that psychological and behavioral factors reciprocally and dynamically interact with physical health/illness. Linear causality does not exist in this reciprocal relationship. Instead, behavioral medicine interventions assume that by addressing psychosocial and behavioral factors relevant to the illness in question, the overall clinical picture of the condition will improve.

In the early days of pain medicine, treatments for pain patients were primarily biomedical in nature, targeting specific anatomy, physiology, and neurochemistry to alter nociceptive input. However, the proliferation of behavioral research indicates that a number of behavioral and psychological factors contribute to the experience of pain, particularly chronic cases, which has prompted the application of behavioral medicine approaches to pain treatment.

Complex pain cases, particularly noncancer chronic pain, often require multidimensional conceptualization and treatment. Accordingly, multimodal approaches aimed at reduction of pain and resumption of a productive life are considered critical. Behavioral medicine is generally imbedded in a comprehensive multimodal pain treatment program. One of the most commonly used behavioral medicine approaches for pain is cognitive-behavioral therapy, specifically addressing pain-related cognitions and behaviors. Accumulated research in the past 3 decades strongly suggests that

This article originally appeared in *Medical Clinics of North America*, Volume 91, Issue 1.

This work was supported by Grant No. AR48888 from the National Institutes of Arthritis, Musculoskeletal, and Skin Diseases to the first author.

[a] Pain Research and Management Center, Department of Anesthesiology, University of Utah, 615 Arapeen Drive, Suite 200, Salt Lake City, UT 84108, USA

[b] Student Affairs, University of Utah, A Ray Olpin Union Building, 200 South Central Campus Drive, Room 270, Salt Lake City, UT 84132, USA

* Corresponding author.

E-mail address: akiko.okifuji@hsc.utah.edu (A. Okifuji).

doi:10.1016/j.cpen.2009.09.001
periopnursing.theclinics.com

multimodal interventions that include cognitive-behavioral therapy modalities is beneficial and cost-effective.[2,3]

Underlying the cognitive-behavioral perspective is the integration of cognitive, affective, and behavioral factors into an overall clinical picture and treatment of pain patients. In the model, each patient is considered as an active processor of external cues that modulates his/her internal state. Psychological variables such as anticipation, avoidance, contingencies of reinforcement, and mood factors are of particular interest. Clearly, the cognitive-behavioral model is not just patients' responses to actual events, but also learned responses to predict and summon appropriate reactions to actual or anticipated events. The cognitive-behavioral framework assumes that how patients perceive their situation and what they expect from their conditions are significant contributors to their health status and disability.

There are five central assumptions that characterize the cognitive-behavioral perspective on pain management (see **Box 1**). The first assumption is that all people are active processors of information rather than passive entities reacting to events or physical cues. Information is processed through use of well-developed cognitive schemes that people have developed as a result of their learning histories. The process is generally overlearned and automated, and thus people are often not aware that they are operating from a set of assumptions that guide their behavior. Nevertheless, people are constantly engaged in this process in their attempt to make sense of the world around them. People can and do adjust their cognitive schemes to adapt to changing environmental demands.

A second assumption of the cognitive-behavioral perspective is that one's cognitive attributions, beliefs, and expectancies can elicit or modulate affect and physiological arousal, both of which may serve as impetuses for behavior. Conversely, affect, physiology, and behavior can instigate or influence one's thinking processes. This cycle is dynamic and continuous, and a causal direction is less of a concern than awareness that this interactive process extends over time with the interaction of thoughts, feelings, physiological activity, and behavior.

The third assumption of the cognitive-behavioral perspective is that behaviors occur as a function of reciprocal interaction between the environment and the individual. Given an event, people respond to the environment, which may in turn alter the environment and elicit others to behave in certain ways. In a very real sense, people are the most prominent contributors to their environments. The chain of such interactions over time makes each person's behavioral pattern unique and idiosyncratic. Ironically, most people are not aware of this process and make external attributions for their failures and successes. For pain patients, it is important to help them recognize how they

---

Box 1
Basic assumptions of cognitive-behavioral treatment

1. People are active processors of information rather than passive reactors to environmental contingencies.

2. Thoughts (for example, appraisals, attributions, expectancies) can elicit or modulate physiological and affective responses, both of which may serve as impetuses for behavior. Conversely, affect, physiology, and behavior can instigate or influence one's thinking processes.

3. Behavior is reciprocally determined by both the environment and the individual.

4. In the same way as people are instrumental in the development and maintenance of maladaptive thoughts, feelings, and behaviors, they can, are, and should be considered active agents of change of their maladaptive modes of responding.

influence their environment to increase support and decrease hindrances to treatment success.

The final assumption of the cognitive-behavioral perspective is that people create their own reality. Just as they are instrumental in the development and maintenance of maladaptive thoughts, feelings, and behaviors, they can, are, and should be considered active agents of change. Pain patients can replace maladaptive modes of responding with more adaptive ones. Pain patients, no matter how severe their pain and despite their common beliefs to the contrary, are not helpless pawns of fate. They can and should become instrumental in learning and carrying out more effective modes of responding to their environment and their situation.

BEHAVIORAL MEDICINE ASSESSMENT OF PAIN PATIENTS

The main vehicle of behavioral medicine assessment is a clinical interview with a patient and, if available and feasible, his or her family members. As supplemental informational sources, standardized self-report inventories may be used. The main goals of assessment are to (1) evaluate psychosocial and behavioral factors relevant to the patient's pain and (2) organize and evaluate the relevant information to direct treatment plans. Attention is also given to identification of any factors that might be impediments to rehabilitation as well as factors that may facilitate the rehabilitative processes.

Typically, the assessment protocol consists of three parts. The first part focuses on understanding a clinical picture of the patient's experience of pain. Specifically, a brief history of pain, learning current pain parameters (eg, quality of pain, time parameters, aggravating/relieving factors), other relevant medical history, and assessing current functional levels, including sleep quality and functional impairment due to pain. It is also important to assess how the patient conceptualizes his or her own pain, the patient's understanding of the potential etiological factors, whether he or she believes adequate diagnostic work has been done, and his or her expectations as to what types of treatments may affect adherence to the treatment regimen and ultimately the success of treatment.

The second part of assessment focuses on gaining a broader understanding of the patient. This includes psychosocial history, including family and personal history of pain, functional abilities and limitations, psychological disorders, and problems with substances (including prescription drugs). This information should help the assessor gain a better understanding of how the patient has historically coped with illness and stress, current life circumstances that may aid/impede treatment efforts, and the level of coping resources available to the patient.

The third part of the assessment is a psychological examination to assess the patient's current mental status, mood functions, and any maladaptive behavioral patterns that may influence the course of pain rehabilitation. Because of the high rate of depression and anxiety among pain patients, it is important to address these issues. All of this information is integrated with biomedical information and is used in treatment planning. There should be a close relationship between the data acquired during the assessment phase and the nature, focus, and goals of the therapeutic regimen.

COGNITIVE-BEHAVIORAL THERAPY: SELF-MANAGEMENT OF PAIN

As noted previously, cognitive-behavioral therapy (CBT) is the most commonly used approach in behavioral medicine for pain patients. There are three main components of CBT for pain: patient education, behavioral skill training, and cognitive-skill training.

Patient Education

Since the patient's active participation is critical for successful CBT, it is often essential that patients attain some understanding of the basic psychophysiological processes related to pain, sleep, function, and mood. The difference between acute pain and chronic pain, hurt versus harm concept, and what to expect from rehabilitation processes versus acute pain therapy can set the stage for skill training. Knowledge related to the behavioral principles, such as conditioning, reinforcement, pain/illness behaviors, and how those principles interact with pain and disability can also help patients prepare for the behavioral skills training phase.

Behavioral Skills Training

Relaxation and controlled breathing exercises are especially useful in the skills-acquisition phase because they can be readily learned by almost all patients. Relaxation and controlled breathing involve behavioral manipulation of the autonomic nervous system by systematically tensing and relaxing various muscle groups, both general and specific to the particular area of pain reported by patients. These skills are useful to reduce anxiety and stress responses associated with pain and improve sleep. It is important that patients understand that relaxation is an active process. Many people mistakenly believe that relaxation is a passive process where one rests and avoids working (eg, laying down in a couch and watching TV). Physiological effects of such active relaxation can be easily measured with a fingertip thermometer that tends to indicate a slight increase in finger temperature due to increased blood flow in the periphery during and after active relaxation.[4,5] Furthermore, it provides a simple demonstration to patients that their behaviors can alter their physiological states, and thereby substantiate the credibility of behavioral medicine approaches.

Another behavioral skill that is often used in CBT is attentional training. Attention plays a major role in any perceptual process. The pain experience tends to be exacerbated by increased attention to pain-related somatic signals.[6] Because our attentional resources are limited, by actively directing a patient's attention to nonpain stimuli, the available attentional resources directed toward pain should decrease. This can be achieved by having patients directly engage in overt behaviors (eg, breathing exercises, progressive muscle relaxation) or use mental imageries to situations that are typically ones unrelated to pain. Although imagery-based strategies (eg, refocusing attention on pleasant pain-incompatible scenes) have received much attention, the results have *not* consistently demonstrated that imagery strategies are uniformly effective for all patients.[7] The important component as to whether this intervention is effective seems to be the patient's imaginative ability, involvement, and degree of absorption in using specific images. Guided imagery training is given to patients to enhance their abilities to use all sensory modalities. The specifics of the images seem less important than the details of sensory modalities incorporated and the patient's involvement in these images. Patients also vary in their ability to use distraction techniques as well as what they find to be an adequate distraction target. The collaborative working relationship between a therapist and patient becomes essential during this part of training.

A variety of other behavioral skills training can be incorporated into the treatment plan to meet patients' clinical needs. For example, some patients experience interpersonal stress to be a major aggravating factor for their pain. Interpersonal relationships are a key component of an individual's environment. Basic interpersonal skills training in the areas of communication, assertiveness, and problem-solving skills may help patients better regulate their stress levels and increase their ability to actively manage their pain.

Cognitive skills training

Typical cognitive training for pain management begins with helping patients understand their own cognitive response system. Specifically, patients can learn to monitor situational factors that tend to trigger their pain/stress and what they actually experience emotionally, behaviorally, and physically when they have pain/stress (see **Table 1**). In the middle column, patients monitor and understand their own processes that may mediate the relationship between situational factors and the consequential experience. There are a number of potential processes that can be discussed; however, the focus is on cognitive processes that patients learn to monitor and regulate.

Effective self-regulation of pain depends on the individual's specific ways of dealing with pain, adjusting to pain, and reducing or minimizing pain and distress caused by pain through use of coping strategies. Coping strategies include positive self-talk focused on the intention to manage pain and the belief that one is able to execute necessary acts to do so effectively. Through the use of coping strategies, a person has an improved chance of successfully engaging in everyday activities, thereby reducing functional limitations and enhancing his or her sense of control over pain and associated symptoms. It is, however, important to note that effective coping largely depends on various personal (eg, self-efficacy beliefs), situational (eg, work, living arrangements), and psychosocial factors (eg, family history of pain, level of support). Interaction between coping strategies and personal and situational factors may be a critical factor in how coping strategies are implemented. Clinicians need to understand how patients interpret their world through the use of their cognitive systems (eg, self-talk, self-efficacy beliefs, instrumentality).

In cognitive skills training, self-efficacy beliefs are particularly important in treatment. Self-efficacy is defined as a personal conviction that one can effectively handle a situation by executing a course of action to produce a desired outcome.[8] The self-efficacy expectation is a critical mediator of therapeutic change for chronic pain patients.[9] Pain patients' self-efficacy beliefs are largely influenced by their own past success/failure at performing tasks to manage their pain; thus, it is imperative that a therapeutic process leads to an experience of effective performance. Such experience may be created by encouraging patients to undertake a relatively easy task in the beginning and gradually increasing the difficulty to match the difficulty of the desired behavioral repertoire. This developmental process allows self-efficacy to increase. In short, effective coping behaviors are essentially directed by the individual's beliefs that situation demands do not exceed their coping resources.

Another important aspect in cognitive training is to understand specific patients' cognitive repertoires. Tendency to appraise situations negatively is known to deter

Table 1		
Cognitive behavioral framework for stress/pain management		
Stressors	**Processes**	**Stress Response**
What triggers stress/pain cycle	Modulating processes mediating between stressors and stress responses	What experientially happens to a person in response to stressors • Physiological • Behavioral • Emotional

treatment success.[10,11] Some of the common negative cognitions are listed in **Box 2**. In cognitive training, therapists help patients become aware of their own tendency for negative cognitions, and then to exercise the application of alternative ways of appraising the situations. A large number of self-help books and therapy manuals are available to help patients and clinicians go through the process in a step-by-step manner (eg,).[12–14]

BEHAVIORAL APPROACH TO IMPROVE COMPLIANCE AND MOTIVATION

One of the critical requirements for successful rehabilitation of chronic pain is that patients adopt an active, participatory role in their treatments. Literature repeatedly indicates that multidisciplinary pain care that includes an activating therapy to restore functioning is effective,[2] requiring patients to modify lifestyles to incorporate various physical activities. Such adaptation is often difficult even for healthy individuals; a report to the surgeon general [15] shows that 50% of those who sign up with gyms at the beginning of a year drop out within 6 months. Thus, it is not surprising that pain patients find it difficult to comply with regular physical activity regimens, even with the implementation of CBT to improve coping.

Therapeutic effort to help patients comply with their treatment regimen is of a growing interest. Long-term treatment success depends on regular adherence to recommended self-care regimens for people suffering from chronic pain conditions.[16] Historically, clinicians invest less energy in patients who show little commitment to therapies. However, as we increasingly face issues related to chronic illness that are closely tied with people's lifestyle issues, helping patients comply with functional regimens has become a critical clinical issue in pain management.

Motivation Enhancement Therapy

Motivation Enhancement Therapy (MET), developed by William Miller and his colleagues,[17] is one of the therapeutic methods that targets patient motivation. MET is based on the assumption that people vary in their degree of readiness for change. Stated differently, patients are considered to be in a certain motivational stage of change. MET strategies are organized to help a patient move from a low level of motivation (or a lower level in the model) to increased motivation (or a higher level in the

---

Box 2
Examples of common negative cognitive patterns

Polarizing pattern: Black-and-white thinking. If a patient's performance falls short of perfect, the patient sees himself or herself as a total failure, leading to high expectation that is often unattainable.

Overgeneralization pattern: A patient generalizes beyond the specific facts of a situation, and sees a single negative experience as a never-ending pattern of defeat.

Catastrophizing pattern: A patient consistently assumes the worst possible outcomes. The patient's understanding of his or her own plight is extremely negative and the patient tends to interpret relatively minor problems as major catastrophes.

Filtering pattern: A patient focuses on a single negative detail, rather than a whole picture, of the event and lets the single detail characterize the entire experience.

Emotional reasoning pattern: A patient assumes that his or her negative emotions reflect the reality. "I really feel it, therefore this must be true."

model) via therapist-patient interactions. Each of the motivational stages is presented in **Box 3**.

MET is a problem-focused, therapist-directed approach aiming to help patients enhance their commitment and motivation for treatment. MET offers a collection of therapeutic techniques to help patients (1) clearly recognize their problems, (2) perform a personal cost-benefit analysis of their therapeutic or countertherapeutic behaviors, (3) develop consistency between their therapy goals and motivation, and (4) internalize motivational thoughts via improved self-efficacy.

MET has been tested for facilitating change to reduce problem behaviors, such as smoking,[18,19] problem drinking,[20,21] problem gambling,[22] eating disorders [23] and high risk sexual behaviors.[24,25] MET has also been shown to increase healthy behaviors such as promoting exercise with myocardial infarction patients,[26] adherence to glucose control regimen in patients with diabetes,[27] and mammography screening.[28]

Motivation Enhancement Therapy for Pain Patients

MET is based on the assumption that people vary in their levels of commitment and motivation for complying with activating regimens. There are several key components in MET [29] that facilitate increased motivation to change maladaptive behavioral patterns and replace them with more adaptive ones. First, a clinician should refrain from judgmental attitudes and responses. Empathy and reflection of patients' feelings is useful at the early stage of MET. Rolling with resistance (ie, not pressuring the patient to change) is another essential interpersonal strategy used in MET. The clinician and patient should remain on the same side, thereby not increasing resistance to change. One of the easy pitfalls is for a clinician to push his or her agenda and as a consequence, let the patient present a counter-argument for why he or she should not engage in therapeutic effort. By going with the patient's resistance, the clinician facilitates the formation of a therapeutic alliance, which is critical to increase the patient's motivation to change. Second, the clinician helps patients to identify specific discrepancies between what they want from pain care (eg, "I want to get well and go out more often") and what they actually do (eg, "I can't do my exercise because I have no time and I don't feel well"). By focusing on the discrepancy, patients gain insight that their maladaptive behaviors and attitudes are actually preventing them from obtaining their goal of getting better. This insight promotes the patient's motivation to change. Similarly, patients benefit greatly from engaging in "decisional balance analysis" of their own behaviors. For example, patients list their "pros" for exercising, as well as for not exercising, and "cons" for exercising as well as for not exercising, which can be discussed and used to increase the discrepancy between the patient's goals and actions. The

---

Box 3
Stages of change

1. **Precontemplative stage:** Patient does not perceive a need to change and actively resists change.

2. **Contemplation stage:** Patient begins to see a need for change and may consider making a change in the future

3. **Preparation stage:** Patient feels ready to change and takes a first concrete (behavioral) change

4. **Action stage:** Patient actively engages in behaviors consistent with regimen

5. **Maintenance stage:** Patient executes plans to sustain the changes made

decisional balance analysis helps patients gain a better understanding of their behavior, in this case, why they do not want to exercise. Through this process, patients become more aware of their role in maintaining maladaptive behaviors as well as identifying strategies to engage in more adaptive behaviors.

Another essential feature of MET is to provide a supportive environment to nurture a sense of self-efficacy and ultimately a patient's ability to change his or her behaviors. By understanding that change is a process that the patient has control over, patients realize that change is possible. With increased self-efficacy beliefs comes a sense of responsibility and an awareness that it is patients themselves who will choose to engage in therapeutic efforts and execute them. MET is a clinician-directed approach that is heavily patient-centered. Detailed descriptions of the specific MET approach are beyond the scope of this paper. Interested readers may find a comprehensive book by Miller and Rollnick helpful.[29]

SUMMARY

Managing pain patients can be a challenging task for many clinicians because of the complexity of the condition. Pain by definition [30] is a multifactorial phenomenon for which biomedical factors interact with a web of psychosocial and behavioral factors. Behavioral medicine approaches for pain generally address specific cognitive and behavioral factors relevant to pain, thereby aiming to modify the overall pain experience and help restore functioning and quality of life in pain patients.

Behavioral medicine focuses on patients' motivation to comply with a rehabilitative regimen, particularly those with chronic, disabling pain. Since patients' own commitment and active participation in a therapeutic program are critical for the successful rehabilitation, the role that behavioral medicine can play is significant. It is not unreasonable to state that success outcomes of the rehabilitative approach depend on how effectively behavioral medicine can be integrated into the overall treatment plan. Past research in general supports this assertion, demonstrating clinical benefit and cost-effectiveness of multidisciplinary interventions that include behavioral medicine. Some of the approaches listed in this paper can be incorporated into clinicians' practice regardless of specialties, and such practice will likely provide helpful venues for managing pain patients.

REFERENCES

1. Gentry WD. Behavioral medicine: A new research paradigm. In: Gentry WD, editor. Handbook of behavioral medicine. New York: Guilford; 1984.
2. Okifuji A. Interdisciplinary pain management with pain patients: evidence for its effectiveness. Sem Pain Med 2003;1(2):110–9.
3. Turk DC. Clinical effectiveness and cost-effectiveness of treatments for patients with chronic pain. Clin J Pain 2002;18(6):355–65.
4. Bacon M, Poppen R. A behavioral analysis of diaphragmatic breathing and its effects on peripheral temperature. J Behav Ther Exp Psychiatry 1985;16(1): 15–21.
5. Jacobson AM, Manschreck TC, Silverberg E. Behavioral treatment for Raynaud's disease: a comparative study with long-term follow-up. Am J Psychiatry 1979; 136(6):844–6.
6. McCabe C, Lewis J, Shenker N, et al. Don't look now! Pain and attention. Clin Med 2005;5(5):482–6.
7. Fernandez E, Turk DC. The utility of cognitive coping strategies for altering pain perception: a meta-analysis. Pain 1989;38(2):123–35.

8. Bandura A. Self-efficacy: toward a unifying theory of behavioral change. Psychol Rev 1977;84(2):191–215.

9. Council JR, Ahern DK, Follick MJ, et al. Expectancies and functional impairment in chronic low back pain. Pain 1988;33(3):323–31.

10. Cook AJ, Degood DE. The cognitive risk profile for pain: development of a self-report inventory for identifying beliefs and attitudes that interfere with pain management. Clin J Pain 2006;22(4):332–45.

11. Tota-Faucette ME, Gil KM, Williams DA, et al. Predictors of response to pain management treatment. The role of family environment and changes in cognitive processes. Clin J Pain 1993;9(2):115–23.

12. Caudill-Slosberg M. Managing pain before it manages you. Revised edition. New York: Guilford Press; 2001.

13. Thorn B. Cognitive therapy for chronic pain: a step-by-step guide. New York: Guilford Press; 2004.

14. Turk DC, Winter F. The pain survival guide: how to reclaim your life. Washington, DC: American Psychological Association; 2005.

15. US Department of Health and Human Services. Physical activity and health: a report of the Surgeon General. Atlanta (GA): Centers for Disease Control and Prevention, National Center for Chronic Disease Prevention; 1996.

16. Turk DC, Rudy TE. Neglected topics in the treatment of chronic pain patients—relapse, noncompliance, and adherence enhancement. Pain 1991; 44(1):5–28.

17. Miller W. Motivational interviewing with problem drinkers. Behav Psychother 1983; 11:147–72.

18. Town GI, Fraser P, Graham S, et al. Establishment of a smoking cessation programme in primary and secondary care in Canterbury. N Z Med J 2000; 113(1107):117–9.

19. Velasquez MM, Hecht J, Quinn VP, et al. Application of motivational interviewing to prenatal smoking cessation: training and implementation issues. Tob Control 2000;9(Suppl 3):III36–40.

20. Brown RL, Saunders LA, Bobula JA, et al. Remission of alcohol disorders in primary care patients. Does diagnosis matter? J Fam Pract 2000;49(6):522–8.

21. Handmaker NS, Miller WR, Manicke M. Findings of a pilot study of motivational interviewing with pregnant drinkers. J Stud Alcohol 1999;60(2):285–7.

22. Hodgins DC, Currie SR, el-Guebaly N. Motivational enhancement and self-help treatments for problem gambling. J Consult Clin Psychol 2001;69(1):50–7.

23. Feld R, Woodside DB, Kaplan AS, et al. Pretreatment motivational enhancement therapy for eating disorders: a pilot study. Int J Eat Disord 2001;29(4):393–400.

24. Carey MP, Braaten LS, Maisto SA, et al. Using information, motivational enhancement, and skills training to reduce the risk of HIV infection for low-income urban women: a second randomized clinical trial. Health Psychol 2000;19(1):3–11.

25. Kalichman SC, Cherry C, Browne-Sperling F. Effectiveness of a video-based motivational skills-building HIV risk- reduction intervention for inner-city African American men. J Consult Clin Psychol 1999;67(6):959–66.

26. Song R, Lee H. Managing health habits for myocardial infarction (MI) patients. Int J Nurs Stud 2001;38(4):375–80.

27. Smith DE, Heckemeyer CM, Kratt PP, et al. Motivational interviewing to improve adherence to a behavioral weight-control program for older obese women with NIDDM. A pilot study. Diabetes Care 1997;20(1):52–4.

28. Bernstein J, Mutschler P, Bernstein E. Keeping mammography referral appointments: motivation, health beliefs, and access barriers experienced by older minority women. J Midwifery Womens Health 2000;45(4):308–13.

29. Miller W, Rollnick S. Motivational interviewing: preparing people for change. 2nd edition. New York: Guilford Press; 2002.

30. International Association for the Study of Pain. Classification of chronic pain. Descriptions of chronic pain syndromes and definitions of pain terms. Pain 1986;3:S217.

The Diagnostic Workup of Patients with Neuropathic Pain

Steven H. Horowitz, MD[a,b],*

KEY WORDS

• Neuropathic pain • Pain receptors • Nervous system

Current concepts of acute and chronic pain disorders distinguish "nociceptive," "inflammatory," "functional," and "neuropathic" pains.[1] Nociceptive pain is the common pain experienced from trauma, cancer, and so forth in which pain receptors (nociceptors) are activated. Transduction, conduction, and transmission of nociceptor activity to a conscious level involves peripheral and central nervous system pain pathways, which, when intact, function in a protective and adaptive manner.[1] However, damage to, or dysfunction of, these pain pathways, peripherally or centrally, can result in a different, much less frequent, but nevertheless important pain picture—that of neuropathic pain.

Neuropathic pain is not a disease in and of itself, but rather a manifestation of multiple and varied disorders affecting the nervous system, particularly its somatosensory components. They include polyneuropathies such as those secondary to diabetes mellitus, alcoholism, and amyloidosis; idiopathic small-fiber neuropathy; hereditary neuropathies; mononeuropathies such as trigeminal, glossopharyngeal, and post-herpetic neuralgias; entrapment neuropathies; and traumatic nerve injuries producing complex regional pain syndrome (CRPS) type II. CRPS type I is also considered a neuropathic pain disorder, although evidence for nerve damage as the underlying mechanism is more controversial. Neuropathic pain can occur in central nervous system disorders, especially spinal cord injury, multiple sclerosis, and cerebrovascular lesions of the brainstem and thalamus. Neuropathic pain in these conditions confers no functional benefit and may be considered a "maladaptive" response of the nervous system to the primary pathology.[1]

This article originally appeared in *Medical Clinics of North America*, Volume 91, Issue 1.

[a] University of Vermont College of Medicine, Burlington, VT 05405, USA
[b] Department of Neurology, Massachusetts General Hospital, 55 Fruit Street, Boston, MA 02114, USA
* Corresponding author. Department of Neurology, Massachusetts General Hospital, 55 Fruit Street, Boston, MA 02114
E-mail address: shhorowitz@partners.org

Unfortunately, the diagnosis of neuropathic pain is often problematic. Clinically, a distinction between nociceptive and neuropathic types of pain is not precise and conditions such as diabetes mellitus, cancer, and neurologic diseases with dystonia or spasticity can produce mixed pain pictures.[2] As with other pains, the perception of neuropathic pain is purely subjective, not easily described, nor directly measured. Also, pain pathway responses to damage are not static, but dynamic; signs and symptoms change with pathway activation and responsiveness, and with chronicity. Further, the multiplicity of disorders that have neuropathic pain as a component of their clinical presentations makes a single underlying pathophysiologic mechanism unlikely; more than one type of pain, and therefore probably more than one pain mechanism, can occur in a single patient, and some symptoms can be attributed to multiple mechanisms.[2,3] For these and other reasons the current management of neuropathic pain should be mechanistic in approach rather than disease-based.[1] Existing disease-based symptom palliation strategies should be supplemented with "targeted" mechanism-specific pharmacologic management.[4]

HISTORY

Despite these complexities, there are several unique features to the clinical presentation of neuropathic pain that can be used to support its diagnosis and should be sought during history taking. In the case of mononeuropathies secondary to trauma, the severity of the pain often exceeds the severity of the inciting injury. CRPS can follow minor skin or joint trauma, bone fractures, or injections. The pain is stimulus-independent and described as "burning," "lancinating," "electric shock–like," "jabbing," or "cramping"; it is often accompanied by pins-and-needles sensations and sometimes by intractable itching (these are considered positive symptoms). These symptoms don't adhere to specific peripheral nerve distributions and often begin and remain most pronounced distally. The pain may be worse at night or during cold, damp weather, and is exacerbated by movement of the affected limb. Multiple types of pain (constant pain with paroxysms and stimulus-evoked pains) can be experienced simultaneously. It is useful to separate stimulus-independent and stimulus-evoked pains to differentiate ongoing from provoked activities.[3] Spread of symptoms outside the initial site of injury is common; in the case of unilateral pain there may be spread to homologous sites in the opposite limb (mirror pain). Positive and negative (numbness, loss of sensation) symptoms can occur concurrently and can be accompanied by autonomic symptoms. Spontaneous pain, often without complaints of sensory loss, is a feature of the cranial mononeuralgias—trigeminal, glossopharyngeal, and post-herpetic. Of course, location, intensity, and duration of pain are extremely important.

In generalized polyneuropathies, rapid progression solely affecting sensory fibers is more likely to be painful, especially if inflammation and ischemia are prominent pathological features, as occurs in the vasculitides.[2] In painful polyneuropathies, eg, idiopathic small-fiber neuropathy, diabetic polyneuropathy with predominant small-fiber ($A\delta$- and C-fibers) damage, the "burning," "lancinating," "jabbing" pains with pins-and-needles sensations are nerve-length dependent and bilaterally symmetric, beginning distally in the feet. With worsening, symptoms ascend to involve more proximal portions of the lower extremities and may eventually affect the hands. This centripetal progression can also occur in intercostal nerve distributions, beginning anteriorly over the midline of the torso with later symmetric lateral extension to the flanks. Autonomic complaints, eg, abnormal sweating, impotence, orthostatic hypotension, and gastrointestinal symptoms, are frequent.

CLINICAL EXAMINATION

Among the more common and important clinical signs in neuropathic pain disorders are positive sensations: stimulus-evoked hypersensitivities such as allodynia to innocuous stimulation, eg, light touch and cold, and hyperalgesia to noxious stimulation, eg, pinprick. They occur focally in mononeuropathies and distally and symmetrically in polyneuropathies. Various forms of hyperalgesia have been described, including touch-evoked (or static) mechanical hyperalgesia to gentle pressure, pinprick hyperalgesia, blunt pressure hyperalgesia, and punctate hyperalgesia that increases with repetitive stimulation (windup-like pain).[2,3] Paradoxically, these hypersensitivities can occur in areas in which the patient also complains of and demonstrates loss of sensation. There can be persistence of stimulus-evoked pain after the stimulus has been withdrawn (aftersensation) in the same anatomic distributions. As with symptoms, spread of allodynia and hyperalgesia outside the original site of injury is common and may extend to homologous sites in the opposite limb. Focal autonomic abnormalities after nerve injury, especially of sweating, skin temperature, and skin color, in conjunction with the aforementioned pain, fulfill the diagnostic criteria of CRPS (vide infra). With chronicity, trophic changes of the skin and nails develop, as do motor symptoms such as weakness, tremor, and dystonia. Nerve percussion at points of compression, entrapment, or irritation can elicit pins-and-needles or "electrical" sensations (Tinel's sign).

In small-fiber neuropathies, deficits are found in thermal and pain perceptions and sometimes touch, whereas large-fiber functions, eg, muscle strength, reflexes, and perception of vibratory and proprioceptive stimuli, are normal. In combined large- and small-fiber polyneuropathies, all these functions are compromised. Symmetrical distal autonomic dysfunction is often present but rarely severe.

While it is common for there to be relatively modest demonstrable clinical neurological deficits in patients with significant neuropathic pain, in some conditions there may be completely normal clinical examinations. This is the rule in trigeminal and glossopharyngeal neuralgias and it occurs more than occasionally in post-herpetic neuralgia. But some patients, particularly with what appear to be small-fiber neuropathies or specific nerve injuries, who describe their pains with the aforementioned typical neuropathic pain adjectives, also have normal examinations. There is the temptation to attribute their pain complaints to functional etiologies; however, at least from a logical perspective, that cannot always be the case, and if they are known to have a particular disease such as diabetes, or suffered an injury in which nerve damage is likely, pain may be their only manifestation of neural dysfunction. In such situations and, of course, in most cases in which further diagnostic information would be helpful, ancillary testing can be used.

Ancillary Tests

Any consideration of the utility of ancillary tests to support the diagnosis of specific neuropathic pain mechanisms must take into account several factors: (1) Currently, available tests only evaluate nervous system structures and functions presumed to be relevant to pain perception and transmission; from their results the presence, extent, and mechanisms of neuropathic pain are, at best, inferred. This situation is somewhat similar to testing for diabetes mellitus with peripheral nerve, ophthalmologic, and renal studies without the availability of plasma glucose levels. (2) There is a spectrum of clinical and physiological manifestations of neural injury within each disorder, with chronic pain occurring in only a small percentage of affected patients. For example, neuropathic pain occurs in ~16% of patients with diabetes mellitus and a third of those with diabetic neuropathy [5]; post-herpetic neuralgia, defined as chronic pain present 4 or more months after resolution of the acute herpes zoster (shingles) rash, occurs in 13% to 20% of patients [6]; and following direct nerve injury, as occurs during venipuncture, persistent pain is rare, perhaps occurring in 1:1,500,000 procedures.[7] (3) The causes of this clinical variability are less than certain, but the presence of pain is presumed to reflect damage to the small myelinated (Aδ-) and unmyelinated (C-) fibers within peripheral nerves.[2] As these fiber types also mediate other clinical functions that are measurable, eg, appreciation of painful stimuli, temperature perception, and autonomic activity, many tests have focused on demonstrating defects in these modalities to verify Aδ- or C-fiber damage.

Clinical Neurophysiology

Neurophysiologic testing, principally nerve conduction studies and electromyography, are frequently used in suspected disorders of the peripheral nervous system. The usual techniques, with surface electrodes for nerve stimulation and evoked potential recording, measure activity of the largest and fastest conducting sensory and motor myelinated nerve fibers (Aαβ-). The most significant measured parameters are maximum conduction velocity (NCV) for the segment of nerve between the stimulating and recording electrodes, and amplitude and configuration of the resulting signals—the compound motor action potential (CMAP) evoked from motor fibers and the sensory nerve action potential (SNAP) evoked from sensory fibers. For central nervous system or proximal peripheral nerve disorders, somatosensory and magnetic evoked potential studies can be helpful. Electromyography (EMG) is the needle evaluation of muscles and evaluates muscle and motor nerve fiber activities.

Unfortunately, Aδ- and C-fiber activities cannot be tested with these techniques. Slowing in maximum NCVs or loss of CMAP or SNAP amplitudes, indicative of peripheral nerve disease either focally or generally, occur as a consequence of large fiber dysfunction. Abnormal EMG features such as acute and chronic denervation indicate involvement of large motor nerve fibers, also focally or generally, from the anterior horn cell distally. If present in a patient with neuropathic pain, these abnormalities can be used to corroborate the clinical impression of damage to a specific peripheral nerve or to peripheral nerves in general as in a polyneuropathy, eg, diabetic or alcoholic neuropathy. However, polyneuropathies or focal nerve lesions with only small-fiber involvement can have normal NCVs and EMG despite significant nerve damage and neuropathic pain.

Quantitative Sensory Testing

Quantitative sensory testing (QST) is used with increasing frequency, especially in clinical therapeutic trials, and measures sensory thresholds for pain, touch, vibration, and hot and cold temperature sensations. A number of devices are commercially available and range from handheld tools to sophisticated computerized equipment with complicated testing algorithms, standardization of stimulation and recording procedures, and comparisons to age- and gender-matched control values. With this technology, specific fiber functions can be assessed: Aδ-fibers with cold and cold-pain detection thresholds, C-fibers with heat and heat-pain detection thresholds, and large fiber (Aαβ-) functions with vibration detection thresholds. Elevated sensory thresholds correlate with sensory loss and lowered thresholds occur in allodynia and hyperalgesia.[8] In a generalized polyneuropathy when all quantitative sensory thresholds are elevated, it is inferred that all fiber types are affected, whereas if a dissociation exists wherein vibration thresholds are normal, but the other thresholds are elevated, the presence of a small-fiber neuropathy is suspected. In asymptomatic patients, abnormal QST thresholds suggest subclinical nerve damage.

The advantages of quantitation of sensory perception are that by enumerating an individual patient's findings and comparing them with normative values a clearer distinction between normal and abnormal responses occurs, thereby allowing analyses across patient and disease groups and for baseline standards in longitudinal studies. However, it must be appreciated that QST is a psychophysical test and therefore is dependent upon patient motivation, alertness, and concentration. Patients can willingly perform poorly, and even when not doing so there are large intra- and interindividual variations. Further, abnormal findings are not specific for peripheral nerve dysfunction; central nervous system disorders will also affect sensory thresholds.

Autonomic Function Testing

The evaluation of autonomic functions in patients suspected of having neuropathic pain can be important because of anatomic similarities between pain and autonomic fibers outside the central nervous system (CNS), and because disorders productive of neuropathic pain frequently have signs and symptoms of autonomic dysfunction (dry eyes or mouth, skin temperature and color changes, sweating abnormalities, orthostatic hypotension, heart rate responses to deep breathing, edema, and so forth). The majority of autonomic tests study skin temperature, and sudomotor, baroreceptor, vasomotor, and cardiovagal functions; they have been extensively reviewed.[9,10] A semiquantitative composite autonomic symptoms score (CASS), composed of the results of sudomotor, cardiovagal, and adrenergic testing, has been devised.[11] Less frequently, pupillary, gastrointestinal, and sexual function tests are helpful.

The value of autonomic testing in patients with a general neuropathic pain disorder, painful small-fiber neuropathy with burning feet, has been illustrated in several studies [12,13] in which many patients had normal or only mildly abnormal electrophysiologic (NCVs/EMG) findings. Autonomic abnormalities were seen in more than 90% of patients, the most useful tests being the quantitative sudomotor axon reflex test (QSART), thermoregulatory sweat test, heart rate responses to deep breathing, Valsalva ratio, and surface skin temperature.[12,13] However, in a recent study of patients with diabetic polyneuropathy, discordance was noted between efferent C-fiber responses in sudomotor tests (QSART and sweat imprint), and primary afferent (nociceptor) C-fiber axon-reflex flare responses. These findings indicate that these two C-fiber subclasses can be differentially affected in diabetic small fiber polyneuropathy. There may be involvement of one subclass and not the other or there may be different patterns of regeneration and reinnervation.[14] Autonomic functions can also be abnormal in peripheral neuropathies not associated with pain.

The relationship between autonomic dysfunction and pain is more complicated in CRPS in which focal sudomotor and vasomotor abnormalities are thought to be essential for the diagnosis [15] and sympathetic blockade has been a mainstay of diagnosis and therapy for decades. As would be expected, the vast majority of patients with CRPS were found to have autonomic abnormalities, particularly involving sweating and skin temperature.[16] However, there are patients with identical focal pain, but no clinical evidence of autonomic dysfunction. These patients do not meet the current definition of CRPS and have been termed "post-traumatic neuralgia";[17] their autonomic functions have not been well studied.

Skin Biopsy

For the past decade the histological study of unmyelinated nerve fibers in the skin has grown in importance in the diagnosis of peripheral nerve disorders, both generalized and focal, including those associated with neuropathic pain. When a skin punch biopsy is fixed with certain antibodies, most frequently protein gene product (PGP) 9.5, epidermal fibers can be stained and visualized.[18,19] Epidermal nerve fiber density and morphology, eg, tortuosity, complex ramifications, clustering, and axon swellings, can be quantified [18,19] and compared with control values.[20] A reduced density of epidermal nerve fibers is seen in small-fiber neuropathies,[21] diabetic neuropathy, and impaired glucose tolerance neuropathy,[22] each of which is associated with neuropathic pain. In a subgroup analysis of one such study, the skin biopsy findings were found to be a more sensitive measure than QSART or QST in diagnosing neuropathy in patients with burning feet and normal NCVs.[23] Conversely, disorders with severe loss of pain sensation such as congenital insensitivity to pain with anhidrosis (hereditary sensory and autonomic neuropathy IV; HSAN IV) and familial dysautonomia with sensory loss (Riley-Day; HSAN III) also have severe loss of epidermal fibers, as does a predominantly large fiber neuropathy, Friedreich's ataxia, in which pain is unusual.[18,19] Thus, the loss of epidermal small fibers is not specific for the presence of neuropathic pain.

Additional tests that may be of value in patients with neuropathic pain, particularly in focal pain syndromes such as CRPS, are bone scintigraphy, bone densitometry, and nerve or sympathetic ganglion blockade. Serum immunoelectrophoresis can be helpful in painful polyneuropathies associated with monoclonal gammopathies and acquired amyloid polyneuropathy. Specific serum antibody tests are valuable in painful neuropathies associated with neoplasia, celiac disease, and human immunodeficiency virus.[24]

SUMMARY

Determining the causes of neuropathic pain is more than an epistemological exercise. At its essence, it is a quest to delineate mechanisms of dysfunction through which treatment strategies can be created that are effective in reducing, ameliorating, or eliminating symptomatology. To date, predictors of which patients will develop neuropathic pain or who will respond to specific therapies are lacking, and present therapies have been developed mainly through trial and error.[25] Our current inability to make therapeutically meaningful decisions based on ancillary test data is illustrated by the following:

In a study specifically designed to assess the response of patients with painful distal sensory neuropathies to the 5% lidocaine patch, no relationship between treatment response and distal leg skin biopsy, QST, or sensory nerve conduction study results could be established.[25] From a mechanistic perspective, the hypothesis that the lidocaine patch would be most effective in patients with relatively intact epidermal innervation, whose neuropathic pain is presumed attributable to "irritable nociceptors," and least effective in patients with few surviving epidermal nociceptors, presumably with "deafferentation pain," was unproven.[25] The possible explanations are multiple and outside the scope of this review. However, these findings, coupled with the disparity in C-fiber subtype involvement in diabetic small-fiber neuropathy,[14] and the recently reported inability of enzyme replacement therapy in Fabry disease to influence intraepidermal innervation density, while having mixed effects on cold and warm QST thresholds, and beneficial effects on sudomotor findings,[26,27] when therapeutic benefit was demonstrated,[27] lead one to conclude that the specificity of ancillary testing in neuropathic pain is inadequate at present, and reinforce the aforementioned caveats about inferential conclusions from indirect data. The diagnosis of neuropathic pain mechanisms is in its nascent stages and ancillary testing remains "subordinate," "subsidiary," and "auxiliary" as defined in Webster's Third New International Dictionary.

As a consequence of these difficulties, the recent approach by Bennett and his colleagues [28] may have merit. They have hypothesized (and provide data in support) that chronic pain can be more or less neuropathic on a spectrum between "likely," "possible," and "unlikely," based on patient responses on validated neuropathic pain symptom scales, when compared with specialist pain physician certainty of the presence of neuropathic pain on a 100-mm visual analog scale. The symptoms most associated with neuropathic pain were dysesthesias, evoked pain, paroxysmal pain, thermal pain, autonomic complaints, and descriptions of the pain as being sharp, hot, or cold, with high sensitivity. Higher scores for these symptoms correlated with greater clinician certainty of the presence of neuropathic pain mechanisms. Considering each individual patient's chronic pain as being somewhere on a continuum between "purely nociceptive" and "purely neuropathic" may have diagnostic and therapeutic relevance by enhancing specificity, but this requires clinical confirmation. Thus, symptom assessment remains indispensable in the evaluation of neuropathic pain, ancillary testing notwithstanding.[28]

REFERENCES

1. Woolf CJ. Pain: moving from symptom control toward mechanism-specific pharmacologic management. Ann Intern Med 2004;140:441–51.
2. Scadding JW, Koltzenburg M. Painful peripheral neuropathies. In: McMahon SB, Koltzenburg M, editors. Wall and Melzack's textbook of pain. 5th edition. Philadelphia (PA): Elsevier Churchill Livingstone; 2006. p. 973–99.
3. Jensen TS, Baron R. Translation of symptoms and signs into mechanisms of neuropathic pain. Pain 2003;102:1–8.
4. Smith HS, Sang CN. The evolving nature of neuropathic pain: individualizing treatment. Eur J Pain 2002;6(Suppl B):13–8.
5. Daousi C, MacFarlane IA, Woodward A, et al. Chronic painful peripheral neuropathy in an urban community: a controlled comparison of people with and without diabetes. Diab Med 2004;21:976–82.
6. Jung BF, Johnson RW, Griffin DRJ, et al. Risk factors for postherpetic neuralgia in patients with herpes zoster. Neurology 2004;62:1545–51.
7. Newman BH. Venipuncture nerve injuries after whole-blood donation. Transfusion 2001;41:571.
8. Suarez GA, Dyck PJ. Quantitative sensory assessment. In: Dyck PJ, Thomas PK, editors. Diabetic neuropathy. 2nd edition. Philadelphia (PA): Saunders; 1999. p. 151–69.
9. Low PA, Mathias CJ. Quantitation of autonomic impairment. In: Dyck PJ, Thomas PK, editors. Peripheral neuropathy. 4th edition. Philadelphia (PA): Elsevier Saunders; 2005. p. 1103–33.
10. Hilz MJ, Dutsch M. Quantitative studies of autonomic dysfunction. Muscle Nerve 2006;34:6–20.
11. Low PA. Composite autonomic scoring scale for laboratory quantification of generalized autonomic failure. Mayo Clin Proc 1993;68:748–52.
12. Novak V, Freimer ML, Kissel JT, et al. Autonomic impairment in painful neuropathy. Neurol 2001;56:861–8.
13. Low VA, Sandroni P, Fealey RD, et al. Detection of small-fiber neuropathy by sudomotor testing. Muscle Nerve 2006;34:57–61.

14. Berghoff M, Kilo S, Hilz MJ, et al. Differential impairment of the sudomotor and nociceptor axon-reflex in diabetic peripheral neuropathy. Muscle Nerve 2006; 33:494–9.
15. Merskey H, Bogduk N. Classification of chronic pain: descriptions of chronic pain syndromes and definitions of pain terms. In: Merskey H, Bogduk N, editors. Task force on taxonomy of the International Association for the study of pain. Seattle (WA): IASP Press; 1994. p. 39–43.
16. Chelimsky TC, Low PA, Naessens JM, et al. Value of autonomic testing in reflex sympathetic dystrophy. Mayo Clin Proc 1995;70:1029–40.
17. Wasner G, Schattschneider J, Binder A, et al. Complex regional pain syndrome—diagnostic, mechanisms, CNS involvement and therapy. Spinal Cord 2003;41: 61–75.
18. Kennedy WR. Opportunities afforded by the study of unmyelinated nerves in skin and other organs. Muscle Nerve 2004;29:756–67.
19. Kennedy WR, Wendelschafer-Crabb G, Polydefkis M, et al. Pathology and quantitation of cutaneous innervation. In: Dyck PJ, Thomas PK, editors. Peripheral neuropathy. 4th edition. Philadelphia (PA): Elsevier Saunders; 2005. p. 869–95.
20. Umapathi T, Tan WL, Tan NCK, et al. Determinants of epidermal nerve fiber density in normal individuals. Muscle Nerve 2006;33:742–6.
21. Holland NR, Stocks A, Hauer P, et al. Intraepidermal nerve fiber density in patients with painful sensory neuropathy. Neurol 1997;48:708–11.
22. Polydefkis M, Griffin JW, McArthur J. New insights into diabetic polyneuropathy. JAMA 2003;290:1371–6.
23. Periquet MI, Novak V, Callino MP, et al. Painful sensory neuropathy: prospective evaluation using skin biopsy. Neurol 1999;53:1641–7.
24. Mendell JR, Sahenk Z. Painful sensory neuropathy. N Engl J Med 2003;348: 1243–55.
25. Herrmann DN, Pannoni V, Barbano RL, et al. Skin biopsy and quantitative sensory testing do not predict response to lidocaine patch in painful neuropathies. Muscle Nerve 2006;33:42–8.
26. Schiffmann R, Hauer P, Freeman B, et al. Enzyme replacement therapy and intraepidermal innervation density in Fabry disease. Muscle Nerve 2006;34:53–6.
27. Schiffmann R, Floeter MK, Dambrosia JM, et al. Enzyme replacement therapy improves peripheral nerve and sweat function in Fabry disease. Muscle Nerve 2003;28:703–10.
28. Bennett MI, Smith BH, Torrance N, et al. Can pain be more or less neuropathic? Comparison of symptom assessment tools with ratings of certainty by clinicians. Pain 2006;122:289–94.

Procedural Approaches to Pain Management

John D. Markman, MD[a],*, Ross Hanson, BS[b],
Annie Philip, MD[c], Ankita Agarwal, BS[a]

KEYWORDS

- Pain • Low back pain • Neuropathic pain
- Palliative care

Procedural approaches remain a mainstay of chronic pain treatment despite the many challenges to the study of their efficacy. Rapid, precise delivery of potent local agents allows pain control targeted at neural structures presumed to mediate the experience of pain. When less invasive analgesic modalities provide inadequate relief, these techniques often play a complementary role. The varied mechanisms of action range from reversible blockade with local anesthetics, augmentation with spinal cord or motor cortex stimulation, and ablation with radiofrequency energy or neurolytic agents. Other procedural techniques access intraspinal routes of medication delivery to improve the therapeutic index of an effective drug, or surgically correct nonneural anatomic pathology that impinges on neural structures. Many of the most common approaches are uniquely suited to offer rapid, potent local control of pain with reduced systemic side effects.

Clinical indications for procedural pain management strategies encompass a broad range of conditions from intractable neuropathic symptoms caused by advanced cancer to chronic, noncancer pain involving the spine. Each technique bears specific risks that pertain to its anatomic targets and therapeutic mechanism of action. Consideration of the evidence for the interventions considered raises practical issues common to virtually all procedures for chronic pain: (1) the validity of extending an indication for cancer pain to noncancer pain, (2) the timing and repeated use of a strategy

A version of this article originally appeared in the March 2007 issue of *Medical Clinics of North America*.

[a] Translational Pain Research and Neuromedicine Pain Management Center, Department of Neurosurgery, University of Rochester School of Medicine and Dentistry, 601 Elmwood Avenue, Box 670, Rochester, NY 14642, USA

[b] Translational Pain Research and Neuromedicine Pain Management Center, Department of Neurosurgery, University of Rochester School of Medicine and Dentistry, 601 Elmwood Avenue, Box 238, Rochester, NY 14642, USA

[c] Department of Anesthesiology, University of Rochester School of Medicine and Dentistry, 601 Elmwood Avenue, Rochester, NY 14642, USA

* Corresponding author. Department of Neurosurgery, University of Rochester School of Medicine and Dentistry, 601 Elmwood Avenue, Box 670, Rochester, NY 14642.
E-mail address: john_markman@urmc.rochester.edu (J.D. Markman).

with temporary benefit in the perioperative setting to a chronic pain condition, (3) the impact of neuroplasticity on the development of tolerance to analgesic effect, and (4) the clinical significance of a reduction in pain intensity in the absence of demonstrable functional or benefit. This article traces the rationale and pivotal evidence for some representative, procedural interventions with the aim of helping nonspecialist physicians identify the patients most likely to benefit from these approaches.

HISTORICAL CONTEXT AND GENERAL CONSIDERATIONS

The discovery of the local anesthetic properties of cocaine and characterization of methods for subcutaneous and spinal injection in the late nineteenth century laid the groundwork for today's procedural pain management strategies.[1] These techniques were refined in the early twentieth century and increasingly deployed beyond the operating room by the end of World War II. Anesthesiology-based "nerve block" clinics of that era have given way to an integrated treatment approach to chronic pain that incorporates psychological and rehabilitative techniques.[2]

A revolution in synthetic chemistry has paralleled refinements in neural blockade. The result has been a growing armamentarium of systemic analgesics including acetaminophen, nonsteroidal antiinflammatory drugs, semisynthetic and synthetic opioid analgesics, and the heterogenous group of medications known as adjuvants. Many of the medications in this last group were developed for conditions such as epilepsy and only later found to have analgesic properties in conditions such as neuropathic pain.[3] In a similar way, procedural techniques shown to have temporary benefit in the perioperative setting have been extrapolated to chronic pain treatment. Despite the emergence of myriad pharmacologic and nonpharmacologic methods to treat chronic pain in an interdisciplinary environment, many of these are not well tolerated or do not sufficiently alleviate symptoms.[4] The potential benefit of local and neuraxial approaches is often greatest when pain remains poorly controlled with pharmacologic and nonpharmacologic strategies.

There are few placebo-controlled studies of invasive approaches for the treatment of chronic pain. Factors complicating the study of procedures include the absence of consensus standards for block technique, the ethical questions and patient enrollment challenges posed by placebo-controlled research, limitations to treatment blinding, and the difficulty of quantifying psychosocial variables such as litigation and family support that influence treatment outcome.[5] As a consequence, the procedures developed for pain management have not been subject to placebo-controlled evaluation approaching the scale of newer pharmacologic agents. This limitation is balanced by most procedural techniques and associated drugs having been adapted from the perioperative context where their use is commonplace and the risks are well characterized.[6]

Symptom and disease-based paradigms, rather than a mechanism-based understanding of pain, commonly inform treatment decisions. Drugs such as gabapentin, for which there is strong evidence of analgesic benefit in a few neuropathic conditions, are routinely used to treat related symptom patterns.[7] Extrapolation of clinical trial data and individualized assessment of treatment response seems to be the norm in pharmacologic and procedural decision-making alike.[8] For example, spinal cord stimulation is used to treat intractable lower extremity chronic pain characterized as "burning" following laminectomy and for a similar symptom characterization in complex regional pain syndrome (CRPS).[9,10] There is no evidence that these symptom patterns share a common underlying mechanism despite the similar features. Patients undergo a defined trial of neuroaugmentation with different configurations of stimulation just as they might engage in a titrated trial of a medication such as gabapentin.

Treatment response, however defined, is not tantamount to a precise disclosure of the underlying pathophysiology of pain. Maximizing the analgesic benefit of procedural approaches requires careful psychosocial assessment of factors that modulate pain intensity and a precise neurologic diagnosis.

The diagnostic role of neural blockade is often overshadowed by its potential therapeutic benefit. The reversible interruption of neural conduction with local anesthetic may be used to disclose the localization and relative contribution of different structures along the nociceptive pathways that mediate the experience of pain. To some extent, this role has increased in importance because the widespread use of detailed imaging studies such as magnetic resonance imaging (MRI) and computed tomography (CT) are sensitive and specific for anatomic changes but not for the presence of pain.[11] This problem is magnified when correlation of imaging with patient report of symptoms is poor. Neural blockade may help determine a peripheral source of pain from a neuroma or entrapped nerve not amenable to visualization with advanced techniques. Blockade may assist in differentiating a local site of pain from a knee joint from that referred in a dermatomal distribution caused by lumbar root injury. Alternatively, regional anesthetic techniques may distinguish somatic from visceral pain as in certain pelvic pain syndromes. There are limitations to the diagnostic value of local anesthetic blockade for localization of chronic pain of spinal origin. For example, attempts to enrich study cohorts for the treatment of facet syndrome with diagnostic blocks have been hampered by low sensitivity and specificity.[12] Repetition of diagnostic blocks and the controversial use of sham blocks in the setting of clinical trials have been shown to improve sensitivity and specificity.[13]

INTRASPINAL OPIOID DELIVERY

Since the 1970s, when endogenous opioids and opioid receptors in the dorsal horn of the spinal cord were first identified, attempts have been made to optimize this form of therapy by delivering opioids centrally. In the few patients with cancer for whom oral and systemic opioid medication does not provide adequate pain control despite opioid rotation, changing the route of administration may enhance efficacy and minimize systemic side effects.[14,15] The principal benefit of intraspinal delivery seems to be the reduction in opioid side effects rather than improved analgesia.[16] Adoption of these approaches has increased in the past 2 decades; as many as 20% of patients with cancer were treated with spinal opioids in 1 series.[17] In patients with cancer, the timing of intervention is among the most difficult clinical questions. Intolerance to systemic opioids, poorly controlled incident pain with movement, and intractable pain caused by neuroinvasive lesions such as involvement of a plexus are among the most common indications. The evidence for the use of these approaches in cancer pain is far more robust than for chronic noncancer pain, in which the risk-benefit balance may become less favorable.

There are many variations of the delivery systems that introduce medication into the epidural and intrathecal spaces, including programmable, implanted pumps, implanted accessible reservoir systems, and tunneled, exteriorized catheters.[18] Epidural and external pump strategies have the greatest value when life expectancy is short (ie, weeks to <2 months). The type of trial that should precede implantation of a permanent device remains an unsettled issue and considerable variation in practice persists. In addition to morphine, which was until recently the only agent approved by the US Food and Drug Administration, dilute local anesthetic preparations and clonidine have been used effectively to augment analgesia.[19] The synergistic effects may confer greater relief in patients with poorly controlled, incident pain and neuropathic pain.[20] Intrathecal ziconotide, a selective N-type voltage-sensitive Ca^{2+} channel-blocking agent, has recently demonstrated a significant reduction in pain in patients with cancer or acquired immune deficiency syndrome.[21] Intraspinal delivery systems enable logarithmic scale reductions in medication dosing but require close monitoring of patients, especially early in the titration phases. The care of patients with tunneled subcutaneous catheters involves routine prophylactic measures (eg, bacterial filters, exit-site care) and monitoring for infection.

The preponderance of evidence supporting intraspinal opioid delivery is based on nonrandomized, uncontrolled series.[22] Two large studies have demonstrated improved analgesic efficacy and reduced toxic side effects in patients requiring high dose of oral morphine.[23,24] The largest randomized prospective clinical trial compared an implantable drug delivery system with comprehensive medical management (CMM) for refractory cancer pain (eg, visual analogue scale [VAS] pain score ≥ 5 on a 0–10 scale). Clinical success was defined as 20% or more reduction in VAS scores, or equivalent analgesia with a 20% or more reduction in opioid toxicity. Sixty of the 71 patients (84.5%) in the intraspinal treatment group achieved clinical success compared with 51 of 72 CMM patients. There was a significant reduction in fatigue and depressed level of consciousness in patients receiving intrathecal therapy. Limitations of this study include the absence of controls for radiotherapy and chemotherapy, younger age of the participants relative to the typical cancer population, and an inconsistent comparative benefit of the intrathecal route of delivery at different time points during the trial. Tight adherence to the algorithm for CMM in the setting of a clinical trial produced a marked improvement in pain control. In a separate small, brief, double-blind, crossover study of epidural and subcutaneous morphine, there was an advantage with regard to analgesia and a reduction in dose and side effects compared with oral morphine.[25]

Lack of validated criteria for selection of patients and long-term data to evaluate the efficacy of intrathecal drug delivery systems in chronic, noncancer pain have limited adoption of this technology. Patients with multiple types of intractable pain with nociceptive and neuropathic mechanisms inferred are described as the candidates most likely to benefit, but investigators who report treatment success in most cases concede patient selection remains difficult.[26] Kumar and colleagues' series[27] reports significant opioid dose escalation with reduced analgesic benefit at 2 years. Favorable retrospective evidence from 12-month follow-up was seen in a small series of patients receiving intrathecal hydromorphone. In 1 study, pump recipients demonstrated improvements in pain, mood, and function from baseline to 3 years following implant.[28] Despite this apparent benefit, these patients experienced a decline in function, an increase in self-rated pain, and endorsed more mood disturbances compared with new patients referred to a pain specialist's practice. This finding suggests that pain severity remains high in these patients despite the intervention. Uncontrolled studies with open follow-up have suggested benefit from long-term intrathecal treatment of spasticity and spasm-related pain with baclofen, a γ-aminobutyric acid (GABA) agonist.[29]

The risks and costs of intraspinal opioids exceed those of systemic opioids. The most common catheter-related problems, occurring in up to 25% of patients, include kinking, obstruction, disconnection, and granuloma formation at the catheter tip with prolonged, high-rate infusion. Retrospective studies have shown the incidence of delayed respiratory depression with intrathecal narcotics to be 4% to 7% and with epidural infusion to be 0.25% to 0.5%. Pruritis occurs in up to 20% of patients and urinary retention in as many as 15%. In 1 series of epidural delivery where nearly three-quarters of patients achieved satisfactory relief, the investigators cautioned that the benefit was offset by the rate of deep infection, including epidural abscess, which reached 13% of patients.[30]

NEUROLYTIC BLOCKADE
Celiac Plexus Neurolysis in Intraabdominal Cancer

Pancreatic adenocarcinoma and cancer of the upper abdominal viscera are commonly associated with severe, poorly controlled pain.[31] In pancreatic cancer, the pain is present early in the course of the disease and the prognosis is poor. Upper abdomen pain is mediated by the afferent nociceptive fibers that travel with the sympathetic fibers of the splanchnic nerves arising from T5 to T12 and the parasympathetic efferent fibers that together form the celiac plexus. The ganglia are situated in the retroperitoneal space adjacent to the L1 vertebral body. Since the initial description almost a century ago, focal destruction of this nerve tissue has undergone numerous refinements that have improved safety and efficacy.[32] The approach is reserved for pain associated with life-limiting illness largely because durable benefit in noncancer abdominal pain has not been convincingly demonstrated.[33] As with other procedural approaches in cancer pain management, some experts advocate the early use of these techniques because of superior pain relief, reduction in opioid side effects, and even improvement in quality of life measures.[34] The evidence is strongest for comparable relief with a reduction in opioid side effects.

Neurolytic celiac plexus blockade is the most extensively studied ablative procedure for the treatment of cancer pain. The most commonly used agent is alcohol, 50% to 100%, which provokes an extraction of lipids and precipitation of proteins.[35] Phenol is also used for neurolysis and may carry reduced risk of postinjection neuritis, but higher viscosity makes it more challenging to inject. With either agent, the variable duration of analgesia is typically in the order of months. The block has been performed using surface landmarks, fluoroscopy, CT, and ultrasound guidance. Numerous variations on the percutaneous, bilateral retrocrural approach have been introduced in the past 2 decades, including transcrural, single-needle transaortic, and anterior, transabdominal approaches.[36] Most centers advocate a diagnostic block with a local anesthetic, such as bupivacaine 0.5%, before neurolytic blockade; a favorable diagnostic block strongly predicts analgesia from neurolysis.[37] More recently, endoscopic ultrasound-guided approaches are being pioneered by gastroenterologists that may prove safer and more cost effective.[38]

There is evidence for the analgesic efficacy of celiac plexus neurolysis in intraabdominal cancer pain syndromes. A recent meta-analysis of multiple retrospective and a single prospective trial found a high rate of successful pain reduction regardless of malignancy type.[39] The results of 21 retrospective studies in 1145 patients characterized "adequate" to "excellent" pain relief in 89% of the patients during the first 2 weeks after the block. Partial-to-complete pain relief continued in approximately 90% of the patients who were alive at the 3-month point and in 70% to 90% until death. Wong and colleagues' prospective, randomized, double-blind, placebo-controlled trial in patients with unresectable pancreatic cancer[40] compared neurolytic celiac plexus block and opioid treatment with opioid treatment alone and sham injection. Pain intensity was clearly reduced in patients undergoing celiac plexus neurolysis but a reduction in opioid and improvement in quality of life were not demonstrated. Rates of reduced need for analgesic drugs and fewer opioid-related side effects have been demonstrated in additional double-blind, prospective, randomized trials.[41,42]

The most common adverse effects of blockade are transient local pain at the injection sites, diarrhea, and hypotension. Neurologic complications including lower extremity weakness and paresthesia occurred at a rate of approximately 1%, although paraplegia and transient motor paralysis have occurred after celiac plexus block.[43] Eisenberg and colleagues[39] meta-analysis found nonneurologic complications such as pneumothorax, pleuritic chest pain, hiccoughing, or hematuria occurring at a rate of ~1%.

STEREOTACTIC RADIOSURGERY
Trigeminal Neuralgia

Trigeminal neuralgia (TN) is a debilitating neuropathic pain condition characterized by paroxysmal episodes of sharp, severe pain occurring in 1 or more branches of the trigeminal nerve. Symptoms are commonly induced by innocuous mechanical stimuli such as light touch or eating. Several etiologically distinct conditions have been implicated in the development of TN, including compression by vascular and neoplastic structures, and primary demyelinating disorders. Demyelination, whether at the junction of central and peripheral myelin in the trigeminal nerve or of the primary afferents in the brainstem, likely represents the common pathway for the development of TN, leading to ephaptic transmission whereby innocuous signals carried by Ia fibers may be transmitted to nociceptive fibers.[44] Patients with TN often obtain a robust initial analgesic response with prophylactic use of carbamazepine, which frequently wanes. Second-line medical therapies tend to offer less robust analgesia and diminished reductions in the frequency and number of pain paroxysms.[45] Myriad treatment modalities for pain relief have been investigated in TN, including several procedural approaches. Microvascular decompression (MVD) of the trigeminal ganglion has largely become the mainstay of treatment in appropriate patients with features indicative of vascular compression, although ablative procedures remain important in patients with TN who fail to demonstrate vascular impingement or who may not tolerate MVD.[46] Stereotactic radiosurgery (SRS) represents a minimally invasive procedural approach to the treatment of TN in patients inappropriate for more aggressive treatments.

Focally targeted radiation may be used to ablate the trigeminal pathway using stereotactic approaches. Precise irradiation of the trigeminal pathway became possible with the development of the gamma knife, with treatments for TN typically targeting the sensory root of the trigeminal nerve.[47] The precise mechanism by which radiation disrupts axonal structures is poorly understood, though animal models[48] have demonstrated nonselective, dose-dependent axonal degeneration following trigeminal irradiation. SRS represents the least invasive current procedural treatment of TN, and is typically indicated in patients considered inappropriate for more aggressive approaches. A 2004 review[49] assessing pain outcomes in 2 studies of a combined 337 patients undergoing SRS for TN described complete pain relief rates approaching 75% initially, although this percentage had decreased less than 60% at 2 years. Two-thirds of patients in this review were able to discontinue anticonvulsant therapy also, but fewer then 50% remained pain free off pharmaceutical treatment at the time of last follow-up. A second study by the same investigator[50,51] compared available surgical destructive techniques for the treatment of TN, and described lower rates of complete pain relief in patients following SRS compared with radiofrequency thermocoagulation and percutaneous retrogasserian glycerol rhizotomy (PRGR) up to 2 years, although SRS regained superiority to PRGR at 36 months. An American Academy of Neurology review[45] reported similar findings for SRS, identifying 3 class III studies reporting complete medication-free pain relief in 69% of patients at 1 year, and 52% at 3 years. These results are similar to response rates seen with other ablative approaches to TN, making SRS an appealing option in patients who may not tolerate other techniques.

Complications seem to occur less frequently in SRS compared with other peripheral destructive techniques for TN and include dose-dependent permanent numbness and dysesthesias (9%–16% of cases), loss of the corneal reflex (up to 10%), and, rarely, hearing impairment.[46,49,50] Asymptomatic vascular changes adjacent to the trigeminal nerve have also been identified during open MVD following failed SRS.[49]

SPINAL CORD STIMULATION
Neuropathic Pain Syndromes

The strategy of modulating the nervous system with an electrical stimulus dates to ancient Rome, with Scribonius' observation that the pain of gout could be alleviated through accidental contact with a torpedo fish.[52] Acceptance of the gate theory of pain in the 1960s led to renewed interest in electrical stimulation.[53,54] Gate theory proposed that pain perception was influenced by the balance of firing between small and large neural fibers. Retrograde stimulation of large fibers would provoke nonpainful stimulation, thereby "closing" the gate through adjustment in the level of voltage. Shealy implanted the first spinal cord stimulator for the treatment of chronic pain in 1967.

In spinal cord stimulation, an array of stimulating metal contacts is positioned in the dorsal epidural space. An electrical field is generated through connection of the contacts with a pulse generator and subsequently programmed in combinations of anodes and cathodes. The resulting field stimulates the axons of the dorsal root and dorsal column fibers, leading to inhibition of activity in the lateral spinothalamic tract and increased activity in the descending antinociceptive pathways.[55] Optimal stimulation is achieved when paresthesias overlap with the anatomic distribution of pain reported by the patient.[56] Either cylindrical, catheterlike leads are introduced percutaneously through a needle or flat, paddle-shaped leads are deployed via an open surgical approach (eg, laminotomy or laminectomy). The power source, similar in size to a cardiac pacemaker, is implanted in a subcutaneous pocket and connected to the leads via subcutaneous tunnel. Advances in consumer electronics have resulted in more precise targeting of neuronal stimulation, improved battery life, and smaller device sizes.

Neuropathic pain of peripheral origin and ischemic pain states are currently the most common indications for this therapy. As with other procedural techniques, patient selection is the key to sustained efficacy. Pain associated with a lesion of the nervous system or dysfunction, or so-called neuropathic pain, in a fixed distribution amenable to stimulation coverage is the most basic requirement. Among the most commonly treated syndromes in the United States are chronic radicular pain after lumbar surgery and CRPS.[57] Neuropathic pain arising from lesions of the central nervous system does not tend to respond to spinal cord stimulation.[58] A temporary trial of stimulation, most commonly performed with percutaneous lead placement, is used to identify patients who might benefit from this approach. Accepted end points for trial stimulation include 50% reduction in pain intensity, patient tolerance of paresthesias, global satisfaction with therapy, and reduction in analgesic medications.[59] The inability to blind patients to the stimulus of spinal cord stimulation in clinical trials, for preimplant assessment, or evaluation of the benefit of permanent placement, is cited as an important limitation to study of this modality.

Two prospective studies of spinal cord stimulation in CRPS have demonstrated statistically significant reduction in pain intensity.[9,60] Harke's study[9] of 29 patients enrolled patients with a prior response to blockade of sympathetic efferents, presumably selecting for patients with sympathetically maintained pain, and demonstrated a greater than 50% reduction in pain disability index scoring. Nearly 60% of patients discontinued oral analgesic medications. An important technical limitation of this study was the high rate of battery replacement (55%) and lead revision (41%). Kemler's randomized study[60] compared spinal cord stimulation and physical therapy in combination to physical therapy alone. At 6 months and 2 years, the mean reduction in pain intensity in the spinal cord stimulation group was greater than 50%. At 3 years there was waning of the benefit of stimulation and statistically significant benefit was no longer observed.[61] Alterations in neuronal connectivity, or neural plasticity, may account for this "tolerance." Three prospective studies of CRPS demonstrated statistically significant reduction in VAS and marked reduction in analgesic requirements.[62–64]

Spinal cord stimulation is used as a late-stage therapy in the treatment of chronic radicular pain after lumbar and cervical spine surgery when other nonpharmacologic, pharmacologic, and less invasive modalities have not provided adequate relief. A prospective, randomized, controlled trial demonstrated superior outcomes with spinal cord stimulation compared with lumbar reoperation.[65] Patients randomized to stimulation were less likely to cross over to the surgical treatment arm (5 of 24 patients vs 14 of 26 patients, $P = .02$) and required reduced amounts of opioid analgesics. The long-term reduction in pain intensity is reported at 50% in a large cohort of patients.[66] A low rate of technical complication in this study was attributed to the development of multichannel devices that seem to limit the need for revision because of electrode migration. Progress in the treatment of the axial component of low back pain with spinal cord stimulation has been reported more recently in 2 prospective trials.[67,68] In both of these studies, the analgesic benefit seems to be more stable in the radicular component. The evidence in refractory angina pectoris is primarily retrospective, but a recent trial demonstrated no advantage compared with percutaneous myocardial laser revascularization with regard to agina-free exercise capacity, and complications were higher in the stimulation group.[69]

The most common complication of spinal cord stimulation across 15 trials ($n = 531$) was lead migration, which occurred in 18%.[70] Infection occurred in 3.7% of cases and battery failure in 3.3%. No studies in the series described earlier reported epidural hematoma or paralysis, but there are reports of both of these complications.

MOTOR CORTEX STIMULATION
Phantom Phenomena

The term "phantom phenomena" describes the complex group of sensory symptoms that often occur following extremity amputations. Phantom pain occurs in 50% to 80% of amputees and includes symptoms of pain and paresthesia, along with awareness and perception of movement in the amputated extremity.[71] The central and peripheral nervous systems demonstrate postinjury pathologic changes implicated in the development of phantom pain. Hyperexcitability of spinal neurons following nerve damage likely plays a central role in the development of phantom pain, as does reorganization of somatotopic mapping in the primary cortices.[71] Spontaneous and aberrant-evoked activity within stump neuromas following axonal injury are seen at a peripheral level, and sensory-sympathetic coupling involving the dorsal root ganglia.[71] Local procedural modalities are less likely to be successful because of the proximal nature of neuraxial pathology in phantom pain, requiring more proximal approaches to symptom control. Motor cortex stimulation (MCS) targets central cortical structures implicated in phantom pain, and may represent a novel approach to treatment of refractory phantom phenomena.

Tsubokawa and colleagues[72] established the potential efficacy of MCS in 1991, demonstrating pain relief following implantation of epidural electrodes to stimulate the motor cortex in 7 patients with thalamic pain. Trials in other pain syndromes and advances in imaging techniques have raised the possibility of expanding the role of MCS, currently used primarily in chronic deafferentation pain refractory to medical therapy. Case series results demonstrating analgesic efficacy observed in the Tsubokawa study have not been reproduced to date. Indications for MCS include brachial plexus, sciatic nerve, and spinal cord injury pain, and phantom limb, post-stroke, and central thalamic pain.[73] Although ongoing research has implicated changes in blood flow in several thalamic nuclei, and the cingulate gyrus, insula, and upper brainstem, it is unclear whether the mechanism of action of MCS is one of facilitation or inhibition.[74] Lefaucheur and colleagues[75] have also demonstrated GABA-ergic neuronal dysfunction and motor cortex disinhibition in hand pain of various causes, suggesting that MCS may work in part by modulating dysfunctional intracortical inhibition.

Following determination of the region of motor cortex most appropriately targeted using MRI, functional MRI, and transcranial magnetic stimulation, MCS electrodes are placed by craniotomy. Intraoperative electrophysiologic testing confirms lead placement relative to the motor cortex, and an electrode is sutured into the dura above the target area with subcutaneous leads tunneled to the skin surface for testing. Electrode leads are tunneled to a subcutaneous pulse generator for long-term therapy following confirmation of efficacy and stimulation territory coverage. Despite advances in imaging and surgical techniques allowing precise lead placement, plasticity in somatotopic organization of the motor cortex still accounts for wide variations in response to MCS.[76]

The largest meta-analysis of MCS included a combined 601 patients from 33 studies of invasive and noninvasive brain stimulation using the VAS to assess the efficacy of MCS on chronic pain symptoms.[77] This analysis demonstrated a weighted responder rate of 45.3% for the noninvasive stimulation group and 72.6% for the invasive group, representing a significant positive effect for both types of treatment. This analysis also found that the number of responders in the noninvasive active group was significantly greater (risk ratio = 2.64) compared with sham stimulation, and that the overall finding of positive effect would be unaltered by the drop-out of any individual study included.[77] Although demonstrating positive findings, this meta-analysis revealed deficits in definition of parameters for stimulation, assessment of duration of analgesia, and variability of disorders among patients. The absence of a sham stimulation control group for the invasive modality arm of the study and problems with blinding were also issues in generalizing results. The meta-analysis suggests that MCS warrants further investigation, but large, well-designed clinical trials to assess efficacy are needed to elucidate the role of MCS in clinical practice. A more recent review included 210 patients undergoing MCS from 14 studies of predominantly central pain.[78] VAS scores demonstrated an average 57% improvement in 41 of 76 patients with available scores. Fifty-four percent of 117 patients achieved good response, as did 68% of the 44 patients with trigeminal neuropathic pain. Despite these results, deficiencies in blinding and the absence of control groups require better-designed studies to support the efficacy of MCS.

Potential complications of MCS stem from typical risks of invasive surgical device implantation and include infection of the surgical site, the implanted electrodes and power source, and intraoperative seizures, epidural hematoma, and subdural effusion.[73] Early postoperative seizures were reported in 19 patients (12%) from 1 review, though none of these patients developed chronic epilepsy.[78]

RADIOFREQUENCY NEUROTOMY
Facet-mediated Spinal Syndromes

Pain of spinal origin is the most prevalent chronic noncancer pain syndrome.[79] There is little agreement among providers as to the role of particular anatomic structures and the underlying pathophysiology of low back pain.[80] The poor understanding of low back pain, lack of accurate diagnostic methods, and difficulty of designing studies to assess treatment efficacy have impeded therapeutic progress for this common problem. Procedural treatments that target specific structures rarely provide complete relief but have been shown to alleviate symptoms when first-line conservative therapies such as medication, rehabilitation, and pharmacologic strategies do not reduce pain intensity and activity limitation. This section considers the evidence for 1 such intervention, radiofrequency ablation, to highlight the complexity and possible benefit of procedural approaches for the complex problem of pain of spinal origin.

The facet joint (or zygapophyseal joint) was localized as the possible anatomic source of low back pain by Ghormley[81] in 1933. The facet joints are paired synovial joints formed by the inferior articular process of 1 vertebra and the superior articular process of the vertebrae below. A tough fibrous capsule is present on the posterolateral aspect of the joint. These small joints are supplied by the medial branch from the posterior ramus of the spinal nerve root. Interest in pain syndromes attributed to the posterior elements of the spine has been overshadowed for much of the past century by radicular localization attributed to intervertebral disc herniation. Large-scale radiologic studies confirm that arthritic changes in these joints were common in asymptomatic patients.[82,83] In 1963, Hirsch showed that pain in the back and upper thigh could be produced by injecting 11% hypertonic saline in the region of the facet joint. In the 1970s, reports of treatment success with radiofrequency denervation of the medial branches revived speculation about the facet joint as a target for the treatment of cervical and lumbar pain.[84] More recent animal models have offered a biochemical basis for the movement-evoked pains attributed to the facet joint.[85]

The diagnostic criteria for facet syndrome remain a matter of controversy. Older age, relief of back pain with recumbency, exacerbation of pain with extension but not flexion, localized tenderness with palpation of the region overlying the facet joint, absence of leg pain, and radiologic characterization of hypertrophied joints have all been proposed as relevant features of "facet syndrome."[86–88] The lack of sensitivity and specificity of these signs and symptoms has complicated attempts to define inclusion criteria for treatment trials. Attempts to define facet syndrome through prospective study of intraarticular facet joint injection have not produced consistent, validated criteria.[89] Intraarticular injections with local anesthetic and steroid have proved to be of little value diagnostically or therapeutically for the treatment of chronic low back pain.[90,91]

Review of the clinical studies of radiofrequency ablation for facet syndrome attests to the difficulty of assessing treatment efficacy in the absence of well-validated diagnostic criteria. Two prospective, double-blind, randomized, controlled trials of percutaneous radiofrequency neurotomy demonstrate lasting relief.[13,92] In both of these trials, patients were enrolled based on response to local anesthetic blockade of the medial branches of the dorsal rami supplying the putatively symptomatic joints.[93] A study by Lord and colleagues[94] achieved a minimum of 50% reduction in pain intensity for 263 days in the active treatment group with cervical zygapophyseal joint pain after motor vehicle accident compared with 8 days in the placebo group. This study applied an uncharacteristically rigorous protocol of 3 blocks (ie, 2 active with differing concentrations of local anesthetic and 1 sham block) to identify patients with zygapophyseal joint (ie, facet) syndrome. Van Kleef and colleagues replicated this result in the lumbar spine with patients selected by response to diagnostic nerve block of the posterior primary ramus of the segmental nerves at L3, L4, and L5. The primary end point of 50% reduction in pain or reduction greater than 2 points on a numeric rating scale was achieved compared with placebo in these patients with at least 1 year of chronic low back pain. The patients undergoing radiofrequency ablation reported a reduction in opioid use and improved Oswestry disability index scores. A third, small prospective trial and a large retrospective series (outcome assessed by third party) demonstrated prolonged benefit in patients with a positive response to diagnostic block compared with nonresponders.[95,96]

Much as in recent large trials of analgesics for neuropathic pain, these positive trial results characterized must be considered in the context of a well-designed trial with a negative result.[97–99] Leclaire and colleague's[100,101] large ($n = 70$), placebo-controlled, double-blind trial in patients with low back pain for greater than 3 months selected by positive response to intraarticular facet injection did not show benefit compared with placebo. The high placebo-responder rates in procedural trials may reduce the likelihood of demonstrating statistical superiority versus placebo, as has been observed in oral analgesic trials.

Others have suggested that the use of intraarticular block by referring physicians may have resulted in greater heterogeneity of the study population (ie, patients whose pain was not truly of facet origin). Such a view highlights the importance of precision in diagnostic injection techniques and interpretation and the broader challenge of matching treatment to patient in chronic pain of spinal origin.

Minor complications from fluoroscopically guided percutaneous radiofrequency ablation occur at the low rate of 1% per lesion site.[102] Localized pain at needle entry site lasting more than 2 weeks was rare (0.5%) and there were no cases of new motor or sensory deficits in this series of 116 procedures (616 sites). Intrathecal injection has been reported in 1 case of chemical meningitis[103] and a separate case of epidural abscess formation.[104]

SUMMARY

Patients who are candidates for procedural approaches are invariably those with the most severe pain. In these patients, procedural approaches to pain treatment offer the possibility of improved pain control through local methods. These interventions do not supplant pharmacologic and nonpharmacologic approaches to chronic pain. Currently, their role is complementary to more conservative approaches, although their success is often measured by the extent to which medication reliance is reduced, particularly opioids. Intraspinal opioids, celiac neurolysis, spinal cord stimulation, MCS, stereotactic radiosurgery, and radiofrequency neurotomy all have demonstrated analgesic efficacy and the potential to reduce the systemic side effects of other therapies. The most challenging aspect of implementing these techniques is matching treatment to individual patient and this is equally true of the many techniques not covered in this article. Diagnostic neural blockade with local anesthetics and temporary treatment trials of stimulation and intraspinal opioids enhance the likelihood of favorable outcomes. As the examination of intraarticular facet injection in low back pain reveals, placebo effect, a favorable natural history, and regression to the mean all may make it difficult to assess the actual benefit of interventions on a case-by-case basis. The study of augmentative approaches further illustrates challenges to establishing meaningful controls and experimental blinding faced by investigators of procedural approaches. Experience is not a substitute for larger, placebo-controlled, randomized prospective trials. Further advances await a deeper understanding of the correlation between symptoms and pain pathophysiology and a more precise understanding of the putative mechanisms of action of procedural therapies.

REFERENCES

1. Katz N. Role of invasive procedures in chronic pain management. Semin Neurol 1994;14:225–35.
2. Bonica JJ. Basic principles in managing chronic pain. Arch Surg 1977;112:783.
3. Markman JD, Dworkin RH. Ion channel targets and treatment efficacy in neuropathic pain. J Pain 2006;7:s38–47.
4. Rowbotham MC. Pain 2002 – an updated review. Seattle (WA): IASP Press; 2002.
5. North RB. Treatment of spinal syndromes. N Engl J Med 1996;335:1763–4.
6. Block BM, Liu SS, Rowlingson AJ, et al. Efficacy of postoperative epidural analgesia: a meta-analysis. JAMA 2003;290:2455–63.
7. Backonja M, Beydoun A, Edwards KR, et al. Gabapentin for the symptomatic treatment of painful neuropathy in patients with diabetes mellitus: a randomized controlled trial. JAMA 1998;280:1831–6.
8. Lenzer J. Pfizer pleads guilty, but drug sales continue to soar. BMJ 2004;328: 1217.
9. Kemler MA, Barendse GA, Van Kleef M, et al. Spinal cord stimulation in patients with chronic reflex sympathetic dystrophy. N Engl J Med 2000;343:618–24.
10. Burchiel KJ, Anderson VC, Brown FD, et al. Prospective, multicenter study of spinal cord stimulation for relief of chronic back and extremity pain. Spine 1996;21:2786–94.
11. Boden SD, Davis DO, Dina TS, et al. Abnormal magnetic-resonance scans of the lumbar spine in asymptomatic subjects. A prospective investigation. J Bone Joint Surg 1990;72:403–8.
12. North RB, Han M, Zahurak M, et al. Specificity of diagnostic nerve blocks: a prospective randomized study of sciatica due to lumbosacral spine disease. Pain 1996;65:77–85.
13. Lord SM, Barnsley L, Wallis BJ, et al. Percutaneous radio-frequency for chronic cervical zygapophyseal-joint pain. N Engl J Med 1996;335:1721–6.
14. Davis MP, Walsh D, Lagman R, et al. Controversies in pharmacotheraphy of pain management. Lancet Oncol 2005;6:696–704.
15. Mercadente S. Controversies over spinal treatment in advanced cancer patients. Support Care Cancer 1998;6:495–502.
16. Mercadente S. Problems with long-term spinal opioid treatment in advanced cancer patients. Pain 1999;79:1–13.
17. Enting RH, Oldenmenger WH, van der Rijt CDC, et al. A prospective study evaluating the response of patients with unrelieved cancer pain to parenteral opioids. Cancer 2002;94:3049–56.
18. Waldman SD, Coombs DW. Selection of implantable narcotic delivery systems. Anesth Analg 1989;68:377–84.
19. Sjoberg M, Nitescu P, Appelgren L, et al. Long-term intrathecal morphine and bupivicaine in patients with refractory cancer pain. Anesthesiology 1994;80: 284–97.
20. Hanks GW, de Conno F, Cherry N, et al. Morphine and alternative opioids in cancer pain: the EAPC recommendations. Br J Cancer 2001;95:587–93.
21. Staats PS, Yearwood T, Charapata SG, et al. Intrathecal ziconotide in the treatment of refractory pain in patients with cancer or AIDS. JAMA 2004;291:63–70.

22. Ballantyne JC, Carwood CM. Comparative efficacy of epidural, subarachnoid, and intracerebroventricular opioids in patients with pain due to cancer. Cochrane Database Syst Rev 2005;(1):CD005178.
23. Smith TJ, Staats PS, Lisa TD, et al. Randomized clinical trial of an implantable drug delivery system compared with comprehensive medical management for refractory cancer pain: impact on pain, drug related toxicity, and survival. J Clin Oncol 2002;20(19):4040–9.
24. Rauck RL, Cherry D, Boyer MF, et al. Long-term intrathecal opioid therapy with a patient-activated, implanted delivery system for the treatment of refractory cancer pain. J Pain 2003;4:441–7.
25. Kalso E, Heiskanen T, Rantio M, et al. Epidural and subcutaneous morphine in the management of cancer pain: a double-blind cross over study. Pain 1996;67:443–9.
26. Kumar K, Kelly M, Pirlot T. Continuous intrathecal morphine treatment for chronic pain of nonmalignant etiology: long term benefits and efficacy. Surg Neurol 2001;55:79–86.
27. Du Pen S, Du Pen A, Hillyer J. Intrathecal hydromorphone for intractable nonmalignant pain: a retrospective study. Panminerva Med 2006;7:10–5.
28. Thimineur MA, Kravitz E, Vodapally MS. Intrathecal opioid treatment for chronic nonmalignant pain: a three year prospective study. Pain 2004;109:242–9.
29. Emery E. Intrathecal baclofen: literature review of the results and complications. Neurochirurgie 2003;49:276–88.
30. Smitt PS, Tsafka A, Zande FT, et al. Outcome and complications of epidural analgesia in patients with chronic cancer pain. Cancer 1998;83:2015–22.
31. Grahm AL, Andren-Sandberg A. Prospective evaluation of pain in exocrine pancreatic cancer. Digestion 1997;58:542–9.
32. Kappis M. Erfahrungen mit localanasthesie bie bauchoperationen. Verh Dtsch Gesellsch Chir 1914;43:87–9.
33. Adolph MD, Benedetti C. Percutaneous-guided pain control: exploiting the neural basis of pain sensation. Gastroenterol Clin North Am 2006;35:167–88.
34. de Oliveira R, dos Reis MP, Prado WA. The effects of early or late neurolytic sympathetic plexus block on the management of abdominal or pelvic cancer pain. Pain 2004;110:400–8.
35. Rumbsy MG, Finean JB. The action of organic solvents on the myelin sheath of peripheral nerve tissue-II(short-chain aliphatic alcohols). J Neurochem 1966;13:1513–5.
36. Cicco De, Matovic M, Bortolussi M, et al. Celiac plexus block: injectate spread and pain relief in patients with regional anatomic distortions. Anesthesiology 2001;94:561–5.
37. Yuen TS, Ng KF, Tsui SL. Neurolytic celiac plexus block for visceral abdominal malignancy: is prior diagnostic block warranted? Anaesth Intensive Care 2002;30:442–8.
38. Abedi M, Zfass AM. Endoscopic ultrasound-guided (neurolytic) celiac plexus block. J Clin Gastroenterol 2001;32:390–3.
39. Eisenberg E, Carr DB, Chalmers TC. Neurolytic celiac plexus block for treatment of cancer pain: a meta-analysis. Anesth Analg 1995;80:290–5.
40. Wong GY, Schroeder DR, Carns PE, et al. Effect of neurolytic celiac plexus block on pain relief, quality of life, survival in patients with unresectable pancreatic cancer: a randomized controlled trial. JAMA 2004;291(9):1092–9.

41. Ischia S, Ischia A, Polati E, et al. Three posterior percutaneous celiac plexus block techniques; a prospective randomized study in 61 patients with pancreatic cancer pain. Anesthesiology 1992;76:534–40.
42. Polati E, Finco G, Gottin L, et al. Prospective randomized double-blind trial of neurolytic celiac plexus block in patients with pancreatic cancer. Br J Surg 1998;85:199–201.
43. Van Dongen RT, Crul BJP. Paraplegia after celiac plexus block. Anesthesia 1991;46:862–3.
44. Wilkins RH. Trigeminal neuralgia: historical overview, with emphasis on surgical treatment. In: Burchiel K, editor. Surgical management of pain. Stuttgart (NY): Thieme Publishing Group; 2002. p. 302.
45. Gronseth G, Cruccu G, Alksne J, et al. Practice parameter: the diagnostic evaluation and treatment of trigeminal neuralgia (an evidence-based review): report of the quality standards subcommittee of the American Academy of Neurology and the European Federation of Neurological Societies. Neurology 2008;71(15): 1183–90.
46. Tatli M, Satici O, Kanpolat Y, et al. Various surgical modalities for trigeminal neuralgia: literature study of respective long-term outcomes. Acta Neurochir (Wien) 2008;150(3):243–55.
47. Kondziolka D, Lunsford LD, Flickinger JC, et al. Stereotactic radiosurgery for trigeminal neuralgia: a multiinstitutional study using the gamma unit. J Nephrol 1996;84(6):940–5.
48. Kondziolka D, Lacomis D, Niranjan A, et al. Histological effects of trigeminal nerve radiosurgery in a primate model: implications for trigeminal neuralgia radiosurgery. Neurosurgery 2000;46(4):971–6 [discussion: 976–7].
49. Lopez BC, Hamlyn PJ, Zakrzewska JM. Stereotactic radiosurgery for primary trigeminal neuralgia: state of the evidence and recommendations for future reports. J Neurol Neurosurg Psychiatr 2004;75(7):1019–24.
50. Lopez BC, Hamlyn PJ, Zakrzewska JM. Systematic review of ablative neurosurgical techniques for the treatment of trigeminal neuralgia. Neurosurgery 2004; 54(4):973–82 [discussion: 982–3].
51. de Siqueira SR, da Nobrega JC, de Siqueira JT, et al. Frequency of postoperative complications after balloon compression for idiopathic trigeminal neuralgia: prospective study. Oral Surg Oral Med Oral Pathol Oral Radiol Endod 2006; 102(5):e39–45.
52. Stillings D. A survey of the history of electrical stimulation for pain to 1900. Med Instrum 1975;9:255–9.
53. Melzack R, Wall PD. Pain mechanism: a new theory. Science 1965;150:971–9.
54. Shealy CN, Mortimer JT, Resnick J. Electrical inhibition of pain by stimulation of the dorsal column: preliminary reports. J Int Anesth Res Soc 1967;46:489–91.
55. Linderoth B, Foreman RD. Physiology of spinal cord stimulation: review and update. Neuromodulation 1999;2:150–64.
56. North RB, Ewend MG, Lawton MT, et al. Spinal cord stimulation for chronic, intractable pain: superiority of "multi-channel" devices. Pain 1991;44:119–20.
57. Alo KM, Holsheimer J. New trends in neuromodulation for the management of neuropathic pain. Neurosurgery 2002;50:690–703.
58. Villavicencio AT, Burneikiene S. Elements of the pre-operative workup. Panminerva Med 2006;7:s35–46.
59. Windsor RE, Falco FJ, Pinzon EG. Spinal cord stimulation in chronic pain. In: Lennard TE, editor. Pain procedures in clinical practice. 2nd edition. Philadelphia: Hanley and Belfus; 2003. p. 377–94.

60. Harke H, Gretenkort P, Ladleif H, et al. Spinal cord stimulation in sympathetically maintained complex pain syndrome type I with severe disability. A prospective study. Eur J Pain 2005;9:363–73.
61. Kemler MA, de Vet CWH, Barendse GAM, et al. Spinal cord stimulation for chronic reflex sympathetic dystrophy-five year follow up. N Engl J Med 2006; 354:2394–6.
62. Calvillo O, Racz G, Didie J, et al. Neuroaugmentation in the treatment of complex regional pain syndrome of the upper extremity. Acta Orthop Belg 1998;64:57–62.
63. Ebel H, Balogh A, Klug N. Augmentative treatment of chronic deafferent pain syndromes after peripheral nerve lesions. Minim Invasive Neurosurg 2004;43: 44–50.
64. Oakley J, Weiner RL. Spinal cord stimulation for complex regional pain syndrome: a prospective study of 19 patients at 2 centers. Neuromodulation 1999;2:47–50.
65. North R, Kidd D, Farrokhi F, et al. Spinal cord stimulation versus repeated lumbosacral spine surgery for chronic pain: a randomized controlled trial. Neurosurgery 2005;56(1):98–106.
66. North RB, Kidd DH, Zahurak M, et al. Spinal cord stimulation for chronic intractable pain: experience over two decades. Neurosurgery 1993;32:384–95.
67. Barolat G, Oakley J, Law J, et al. Epidural spinal cord stimulation with multiple electrode paddle lead is effective in treating low back pain. Neuromodulation 2001;2:59–66.
68. North RB, Kidd DH, Olin J, et al. Spinal cord stimulation for axial low back pain: a prospective controlled trial comparing dual with single percutaneous electrodes. Spine 2005;30:1412–8.
69. McNab D, Kahn SN, Sharples LD, et al. An open label, single-centre, randomized trial of spinal cord stimulation vs. percutaneous myocardial laser revascularization in patients with refractory angina pectoris: the SPiRiT trial. Eur Heart J 2006;27:1048–53.
70. Bennett DS, Cameron T. Spinal cord stimulation for complex regional pain syndromes. In: Simpson B, editor. Electrical stimulation and relief of pain, in pain research and clinical management. Amsterdam: Elsevier Science BV; 2003. p. 111–29.
71. Flor H, Nikolajsen L, Staehelin JT. Phantom limb pain: a case of maladaptive CNS plasticity? Nat Rev Neurosci 2006;7(11):873–81.
72. Tsubokawa T, Katayama Y, Yamamoto T, et al. Treatment of thalamic pain by chronic motor cortex stimulation. Pacing Clin Electrophysiol 1991;14(1):131–4.
73. Brown JA, Barbaro NM. Motor cortex stimulation for central and neuropathic pain: current status. Pain 2003;104(3):431–5.
74. Garcia-Larrea L, Peyron R, Mertens P, et al. Electrical stimulation of motor cortex for pain control: a combined PET-scan and electrophysiological study. Pain 1999;83(2):259–73.
75. Lefaucheur JP, Drouot X, Menard-Lefaucheur I, et al. Motor cortex rTMS restores defective intracortical inhibition in chronic neuropathic pain. Neurology 2006; 67(9):1568–74.
76. Lefaucheur JP, Drouot X, Menard-Lefaucheur I, et al. Neurogenic pain relief by repetitive transcranial magnetic cortical stimulation depends on the origin and the site of pain. J Neurol Neurosurg Psychiatr 2004;75(4):612–6.
77. Lima MC, Fregni F. Motor cortex stimulation for chronic pain: systematic review and meta-analysis of the literature. Neurology 2008;70(24):2329–37.

78. Fontaine D, Hamani C, Lozano A. Efficacy and safety of motor cortex stimulation for chronic neuropathic pain: critical review of the literature. J Neurosurg 2009; 110(2):251–6.
79. Andersson GBJ. Epidemiologic features of chronic low-back pain. Lancet 1999; 354:581–5.
80. Deyo RA, Haselkorn J, Hoffman R, et al. Designing studies of diagnostic tests for low back pain or radiculopathy. Spine 1994;19:2057S–65S.
81. Ghormely RK. Low back pain with special reference to the articular facets with presentation of an operative procedure. JAMA 1933;101(23):1773–7.
82. Magora A, Schwartz A. Relation between the low back pain syndrome and X-ray findings. I. Degenerative osteoarthritis. Scand J Rehabil Med 1973;5:115.
83. Hirsch D, Ingelmark B, Miller M. The anatomical basis for low back pain. Acta Orthop Scandia 1963;33:1.
84. Rees WS. Multiple bilateral subcutaneous rhizolysis of segmental nerves in the treatment of intervertebral disc syndrome. Ann Gen Pract 1974;26:126.
85. Yamashita T, Cavanaugh JM, Ozaktay AC, et al. Effect of substance P on mechanosensitive units of tissues around and in the lumbar facet joint. J Orthop Res 1993;11(2):205–14.
86. Jackson RP. The facet syndrome. Myth or reality? Clin Orthop Relat Res 1992; 279:110–21.
87. Lewinnek GE, Warfield CA. Facet joint degeneration as a cause of low back pain. Clin Orthop Relat Res 1986;213:216–22.
88. Schwarzer AC, Wang SC, O'Driscoll D, et al. The ability of computed tomography to identify a painful zygapophysial joint in patients with chronic low back pain. Spine 1995;20:907–12.
89. Schwarzer AC, Aprill CN, Derby R, et al. Clinical features of patients with pain stemming from the lumbar zygapophysial joints. Is the lumbar facet syndrome a clinical entity? Spine 1994;19:1132–7.
90. Carette S, Marcoux S, Truchon R, et al. A controlled trial of corticosteroid injections into facet joints for chronic low back pain. N Engl J Med 1991;325:1002–7.
91. Jackson RP, Jacobs RR, Montesano PX. Facet joint injection in low back pain. Spine 1988;13:966–71.
92. Van Kleef MV, Gerard AM, Barendse GA, et al. Randomized trial of radiofrequency lumbar facet denervation for chronic low back pain. Spine 1999;24: 1937–42.
93. Resnick DK, Choudhri TF, Dailey AT, et al. Guidelines for the performance of fusion procedures for degenerative disease of the lumbar spine. Part 13: injection therapies, low-back pain, and lumber fusion. J Neurosurg Spine 2005;2: 707–15.
94. Lord SM, Barnsley L, Bogduk N. The utility of comparative local anaesthetic blocks in the diagnosis of cervical zygapophysial joint pain. Pain 1993;18:343–50.
95. Gallagher J, Petriconne di Vadi P, Wedley J, et al. Radiofrequency facet joint denervation in the treatment of low back pain. A prospective controlled double-blind study to assess efficacy. Pain Clin 1994;7:193–8.
96. North RB, Han M, Zahurak M, et al. Radiofrequency lumbar facet denervation: analysis of prognostic factors. Pain 1994;57:77–83.
97. Backonja M, Glanzman RL. Gabapentin dosing for neuropathic pain: evidence from randomized, placebo-controlled clinical trials. Clin Ther 2003;25:81–104.
98. Safirstein B, Tuchman M, Dogra S, et al. Efficacy of lamotrogine in painful diabetic neuropathy: results from two large double-blind trials. J Pain 2005;6(Suppl 3): S34 (Abstract).

99. Thienel U, Neto W, Schwabe SK, et al. Topiramate in painful diabetic polyneuropathy: findings from three double-blind placebo controlled trials. Acta Neurol Scand 2004;110:221–31.

100. Leclaire R, Fortin L, Lambert R, et al. Radiofrequency facet joint denervation in the treatment of low back pain: a placebo controlled clinical trial to assess efficacy. Spine 2001;26:1411–7.

101. Dworkin RH, Katz J, Gitlin M. Placebo response in clinical trials of depression and its implications for research on chronic neuropathic pain. Neurology 2005;65:s7–19.

102. Kornick C, Kramarich S, Lamer TJ, et al. Complications of lumbar radiofrequency facet denervation. Spine 2004;29:1352–4.

103. Thomson SJ, Lomax DM, Collet BJ. Chemical meningitis after lumbar facet joint block with local anesthetic and steroids. Anesthesia 1991;46:563–4.

104. Alcock A, Regaard A, Browne J. Facet joint injection: a rare form cause of epidural abscess formation. Pain 2003;103(1–2):209–10.

Myofascial Pain Trigger Points

Elizabeth Demers Lavelle, MD[a], William F. Lavelle, MD[b],*,
Howard S. Smith, MD, FACP[c]

KEYWORDS

• Myofascial • Skeletal • Muscle

A myofascial trigger point is a hyperirritable point in skeletal muscle that is associated with a hypersensitive palpable nodule.[1] Approximately 23 million Americans have chronic disorders of the musculoskeletal system.[2] Painful conditions of the musculoskeletal system, including myofascial pain syndrome, constitute some of the most important chronic problems that are encountered in a clinical practice.

DEFINITIONS

Myofascial pain syndrome is defined as sensory, motor, and autonomic symptoms that are caused by myofascial trigger points. The sensory disturbances that are produced are dysesthesias, hyperalgesia, and referred pain. Coryza, lacrimation, salivation, changes in skin temperature, sweating, piloerection, proprioceptive disturbances, and erythema of the overlying skin are autonomic manifestations of myofascial pain.

Travell and Simons[1] defined the myofascial trigger point as "a hyperirritable spot, usually within a taut band of skeletal muscle or in the muscle fascia which is painful on compression and can give rise to characteristic referred pain, motor dysfunction, and autonomic phenomena".[1] When the trigger point is pressed, pain is caused and produces effects at a target, the zone of reference, or referral zone.[3,4] This area of referred pain is the feature that differentiates myofascial pain syndrome from fibromyalgia. This pain is reproduced reliably on palpation of the trigger point, despite the fact that it is remote from its source of origin. This referred pain rarely coincides with dermatologic or neuronal distributions, but follows a consistent pattern.[5]

This article originally appeared in *Medical Clinics of North America*, Volume 91, Issue 2.

[a] Department of Anesthesia, SUNY Upstate Medical University, Syracuse, NY 13210, USA
[b] Department of Orthopaedics, SUNY Upstate Medical University, Syracuse, NY 13210, USA
[c] Department of Anesthesiology, Albany Medical Center, 43 New Scotland Avenue, Albany, NY 12208, USA
* Corresponding author.
E-mail address: lavellwf@yahoo.com (W.F. Lavelle).

ETIOLOGY

Trigger points may develop after an initial injury to muscle fibers. This injury may include a noticeable traumatic event or repetitive microtrauma to the muscles. The trigger point causes pain and stress in the muscle or muscle fiber. As the stress increases, the muscles become fatigued and more susceptible to activation of additional trigger points. When predisposing factors combine with a triggering stress event, activation of a trigger point occurs. This theory is known as the "injury pool theory".[1]

PATHOPHYSIOLOGY

There is no pathologic or laboratory test for identifying trigger points. Therefore, much of the pathophysiologic research on trigger points has been directed toward verifying common theories of their formation. **Fig. 1** provides an example of the theory behind the formation of myofascial trigger points.

The local twitch response (LTR) has been described as a characteristic response of myofascial trigger points. LTR is a brisk contraction of the muscle fibers in and around the taut band elicited by snapping palpation or rapid insertion of a needle into the myofascial trigger point[6] The sensitive site where an LTR is found has been termed the "sensitive locus." Based on observations during successful trigger point injections, a model with multiple sensitive loci in a trigger point region was proposed.[6] In a recent histologic study, the sensitive loci correlated with sensory receptors.[7,8]

In a study by Hubbard and Berkoff, spontaneous electrical activity was demonstrated at sites in a trigger point region, whereas similar activity was not found at adjacent nontender sites.[6] The site where the spontaneous electrical activity is recorded is termed the "active locus." To elicit and record spontaneous electrical activity, high-sensitivity recording and a gentle insertion technique into the trigger point must be used.[6] The waveforms of the spontaneous electrical activity correspond closely to previously published reports of motor endplate noise.[9,10] Therefore, the spontaneous

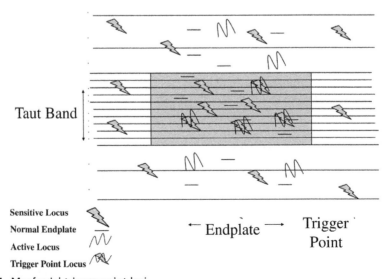

Fig. 1. Myofascial trigger point loci.

electrical activity likely is one type of endplate potential, and the active loci probably are related closely to motor endplates.

It was hypothesized that a myofascial trigger point locus is formed when a sensitive locus, the nociceptor, and an active locus—the motor endplate—coincide. It is possible that sensitive loci are distributed widely throughout the entire muscle, but are concentrated in the trigger point region. This explains the finding of elicitation of referred pain when "normal" muscle tissue is needled or high pressure is applied (**Fig. 2**).

DIAGNOSIS

The diagnosis of myofascial pain is best made through a careful analysis of the history of pain along with a consistent physical examination.[11] The diagnosis of myofascial pain syndrome, as defined by Simons and colleagues,[12] relies on eight clinical characteristics (**Box 1**). Identification of the pain distribution is one of the most critical elements in identifying and treating myofascial pain. The physician should ask the patient to identify the most intense area of pain using a single finger. There also is

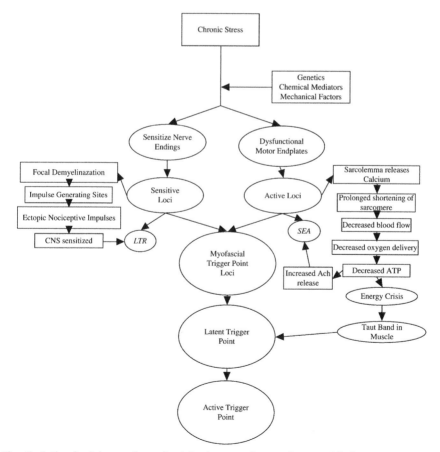

Fig. 2. Pathophysiology of myofascial trigger points. Ach, acetylcholine; CNS, central nervous system; LTR, local twitch response; SEA, spontaneous electrical activity.

Box 1
Clinical characteristics of myofascial pain syndrome

Onset description and immediate cause of the pain

Pain distribution pattern

Restricted range of motion with increased sensitivity to stretching

Weakened muscle due to pain with no muscular atrophy

Compression causing pain similar to the patient's chief complaint

A palpable taut band of muscle correlating with the patient's trigger point

LTR elicited by snapping palpation or rapid insertion of a needle

Reproduction of the referred pain with mechanical stimulation of the trigger point

---

an associated consistent and characteristic referred pain pattern on palpation of this trigger point. Often, this referred pain is not located in the immediate vicinity of the trigger point, but is found commonly in predictable patterns. These patterns are described clearly in *Travell and Simon's Myofascial Pain and Dysfunction: The Trigger Point Manual*.[12] Pain can be projected in a peripheral referral pattern, a central referral pattern, or a local pain pattern (**Fig. 3**). When a hyperintense area of pain is identified, its area of referred pain should be identified.[4]

The palpable band is considered critical in the identification of the trigger point. Three methods have been identified for trigger point palpation: flat palpation, pincer palpation, and deep palpation. Flat palpation refers to sliding a fingertip across the muscle fibers of the affected muscle group. The skin is pushed to one side, and the finger is drawn across the muscle fibers. This process is repeated with the skin pushed to the other side. A taut band may be felt passing under the physician's finger. Snapping palpation, like plucking of a violin, is used to identify the specific trigger point. Pincer palpation is a method that involves firmly grasping the muscle between the thumb and forefinger. The fibers are pressed between the fingers in a rolling manner while attempting to locate a taut band. Deep palpation may be used to find a trigger point that is obscured by superficial tissue. The fingertip is placed over the muscle attachment of the area suspected of housing the trigger point. When the patient's symptoms are reproduced by pressing in one specific direction, a trigger point may be presumed to be located.[2]

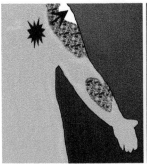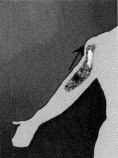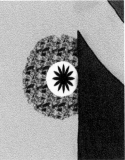

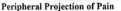
Peripheral Projection of Pain   Central Projection of Pain   Local Pain

Fig. 3. Trigger points and their reference zones.

Several devices have been developed to assist in the location of a myofascial trigger point. Fisher [13] developed a pressure threshold measuring gauge to assist in the diagnosis and location of the myofascial trigger point. It is a hand-held device calibrated in kg/cm^2. Pressure is increased gradually and evenly until the patient reports discomfort. The pressure measurement is then recorded. Contralateral pressure measurements are taken to establish relative sensitivity of the point in question; a difference of 2 kg/cm^2 is considered an abnormal reading.[14] An electromyogram (EMG) also may assist in the diagnosis of the trigger point.[15,16] When the active locus is entered, the peak amplitudes often are off the scale of the EMG monitor. Although this method may seem to be useful scientifically, significant clinical results have not been found.

NONINVASIVE TECHNIQUES FOR MANAGEMENT
Spray (Freeze) and Stretch

Travell and Simons[1] advocated passive stretching of the affected muscle after application of sprayed vapocoolant to be the "single most effective treatment" for trigger point pain. The proper technique depends on patient education, cooperation, compliance, and preparation. The patient should be positioned comfortably, ensuring that the trigger point area is well supported and under minimal tension. Position should place one end of the muscle with the trigger point zone securely anchored. The patient should be marked after careful diagnosis of the trigger point region, and the reference zone should be noted. The skin overlying the trigger point should be anesthetized with a vapocoolant spray (ethyl chloride or dichlorodifluoromethane-trichloromonofluoromethane) over the entire length of the muscle.[12] This spray should be applied from the trigger point toward the reference zone until the entire length of the muscle has been covered. The vapocoolant should be directed at a 30° angle to the skin. Immediately after the first vapocoolant spray pass, passive pressure should be applied to the other end of the muscle, resulting in a stretch. Multiple slow passes of spray over the entire width of the muscle should be performed while maintaining the passive muscle stretch. This procedure is repeated until full range of motion of the muscle group is reached, with a maximum of three repetitions before rewarming the area with moist heat. Care must be taken to avoid prolonged exposure to the vapocoolant spray, assuring that each spray pass lasts less than 6 seconds. Patients must be warned not to overstretch muscles after a therapy session.

Physical Therapy

Some of the best measures to relieve cyclic myofascial pain involve the identification of perpetuating factors. Physical therapists assist patients in the determination of predisposing activities. With routine follow-up, they are often able to correct elements of poor posture and body mechanics.[1]

Transcutaneous Electrical Stimulation

Transcutaneous electrical stimulation (TENS) is used commonly as adjuvant therapy in chronic and acute pain management. Placement of the TENS electrode is an empiric process and may involve placement at trigger point sites or along zones of referred pain.[17]

Ultrasound

Ultrasound may be used as an adjunctive means of treatment. Ultrasound transmits vibration energy at the molecular level; approximately 50% reaches a depth of 5 mm.

Massage

Massage was advocated by Simons and colleagues.[12] Their technique was described as a "deep stroking" or "stripping" massage. The patient is positioned comfortably to allow the muscle group being treated to be lengthened and relaxed as much as possible.

Ischemic Compression Therapy

The term "ischemic compression therapy" refers to the belief that the application of pressure to a trigger point produces ischemia that ablates the trigger point. Pressure is applied to the point with increasing resistance and maintained until the physician feels a relief of tension. The patient may feel mild discomfort, but should not experience profound pain. The process is repeated for each band of taut muscle encountered.[12]

INVASIVE TECHNIQUES FOR MANAGEMENT

Trigger point injection remains the treatment with the most scientific evidence and investigation for support. Typically, it is advocated for trigger points that have failed noninvasive means for treatment. Injections are highly dependent of the clinician's skill to localize the active trigger point with a small needle.

Various injected substances have been investigated. These include local anesthetics, botulism toxin, sterile water, sterile saline, and dry needling. One common finding with these techniques is that, at least anecdotally, the duration of pain relief following the procedure outlasts the duration of action of the injected medication.

THE UNIVERSAL TECHNIQUE FOR INJECTION

The patient should be positioned in a recumbent position for the prevention of syncope, assistance in patient relaxation, and decreased muscle tension. The trigger point must then be identified correctly. The palpable band is considered critical in the identification of the trigger point. This can be done with any of the three methods described above. The trigger point should be marked clearly. Then, the skin is prepared in a sterile fashion. Various physicians use different skin preparations for their local procedures. One common skin preparation technique is to cleanse the skin with a topical alcohol solution followed by preparation with povidone-iodine.[12] A 22-gauge 1.5-inch needle is recommended for most superficial trigger points. Deeper muscles may be reached using a 21-gauge 2-inch or 2.5-inch needle. The needle should never be inserted to the hub because this is the weakest point on the needle.[18]

Once the skin is prepared and the trigger point is identified, the overlying skin is grasped between the thumb and index finger or between the index and middle finger. The needle is inserted approximately 1 to 1.5 cm away from the trigger point to facilitate the advancement of the needle into the trigger point at a 30° angle. The grasping fingers isolate the taut band and prevent it from rolling out of the trajectory of the needle. A "fast-in, fast-out" technique should be used to elicit an LTR. This local twitch was shown to predict the effectiveness of the trigger point injection.[19] After entering the trigger point, the needle should be aspirated to ensure that the lumen of a local blood vessel has not been violated. If the physician chooses to inject an agent, a small volume should be injected at this time. The needle may be withdrawn to the level of the skin without exiting, and it should be redirected to the trigger point repeating the process. The process of entering the trigger point and eliciting LTRs should proceed, attempting to contact as many sensitive loci as possible (**Fig. 4**).

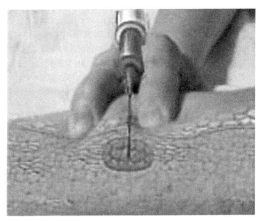

Fig. 4. Injection technique. The trigger point is positioned between two fingers to prevent the sliding of the trigger point during injection. The fingers are pressed downward and apart to maintain pressure and ensure hemostasis.

An integral part of trigger point therapy is postprocedural stretching. After trigger point injection, the muscle group that was injected should undergo a full active stretch.

Complications of Trigger Point Injections

As with the introduction of any foreign body through the skin, the risk for skin or soft tissue infection is a possibility. Injection over an area of infected skin is contraindicated. The physician should never aim the needle at an intercostal space to avoid the complication of a pneumothorax. Hematoma formation following a trigger point injection can be minimized with proper injection technique and holding pressure over the surrounding soft tissue after withdrawal of the needle.[12,20]

MEDICATIONS FOR INJECTION
Local Anesthetics

Local Anesthetics are the substances that have been investigated most frequently for the treatment of myofascial trigger points. Local anesthetic injections were shown to improve measures on a pain scale, range of motion, and algometry pressure thresholds. The volume of local anesthetic injected also has been investigated, and small volumes are considered the most effective. Typically, less than 1 mL of local agent should be injected in a highly controlled manner. The primary use for a local anesthetic is to prevent local soreness. Procaine is selected often because it is selective for small, unmyelinated fibers that control pain perception rather than motor control. Lidocaine is a common substitute for procaine, but no experimental comparisons are available in the literature.[12,21]

Corticosteroids

Local steroid injections offer the potential advantage of control of local inflammatory response; however, the theory that a trigger point is due to a local energy crisis does not support their clinical use. Steroids are used commonly by the orthopedic surgeon and rheumatologist to treat local conditions, such as trigger finger and tennis elbow. They carry the added dangers of local myotoxicity, subcutaneous tissue damage, and skin discoloration.[12]

Botulinum Toxin

Localized injection of a small amount of commercially prepared botulism toxin A relaxes an overactive muscle by blocking the release of acetylcholine. This essentially denervates the muscle until new synaptic contacts can be established. When injecting botulism toxin, the physician should remember that the toxin does not discriminate between trigger points and normal motor endplates. The physician should be careful to localize the trigger point before injection.[22,23]

Dry Needling

Dry needling involves multiple advances of a needle into the muscle at the region of the trigger point. Much like any injection technique, the physician should aim to elicit an LTR, reproduction of the patient's symptomatology, and relief of muscle tension.[7,24]

SUMMARY

Myofascial pain syndromes are a widely recognized phenomenon among physicians and represent a common pain disorder in the American population. A myofascial trigger point is "a hyperirritable spot, usually within a taut band of skeletal muscle or in the muscle fascia. The spot is painful on compression and can give rise to characteristic referred pain, motor dysfunction, and autonomic phenomena".[1] Many treatment strategies, both invasive and noninvasive, have been recognized for myofascial trigger points.

REFERENCES

1. Travell JG, Simons DG. Myofascial pain and dysfunction: the trigger point manual. Baltimore (MD): Williams and Wilkins; 1983.
2. Imamura ST, Fischer AA, Imamura M, et al. Pain management using myofascial approach when other treatment failed. Physical Medicine & Rehabilitation Clinics of North America 1997;8(1):179–96.
3. Maigne J, Maigne R. Trigger point of the posterior iliac crest: painful iliolumbar ligament insertion or cutaneous dorsal ramus pain? An anatomic study. Arch Phys Med Rehabil 1991;72(9):734–7.
4. Sola A, Bonica J. Myofascial pain syndromes. In: Bonica J, Loeser J, Chapman S, et al, editors. The management of pain. Baltimore (MD): Lippincott Williams & Wilkins; 1996. p. 352–67.
5. Long S, Kephart W. Myofascial pain syndrome. In: Ashburn M, Rice L, editors. The management of pain. New York: Churchill Livingstone, Inc; 1998. p. 299–321.
6. Simons D. Single-muscle myofascial pain syndromes. In: Tollison CD, Satterthwaite CD, Tollison J, editors. Handbook of pain management. 2nd edition. Baltimore (MD): Williams & Wilkins; 1994. p. 539–55.
7. Hong C-Z. Trigger point injection: dry needling vs. lidocaine injection. Am J Phys Med Rehabil 1994;73:156–63.
8. Hong C-Z, Chen J-T, Chen S-M, et al. Histological findings of responsive loci in a myofascial trigger spot of rabbit skeletal muscle fibers from where localized twitch responses could be elicited [abstract]. Arch Phys Med Rehabil 1996;77: 962.
9. Simons DG. Do endplate noise and spikes arise from normal motor endplates? Am J Phys Med Rehabil 2001;80:134–40.

10. Simons DG, Hong C-Z, Simons LS. Endplate potentials are common to midfiber myofascial trigger points. Am J Phys Med Rehabil 2002;81:212–22.
11. Graff-Radford S. Myofascial pain: diagnosis and management. Curr Pain Headache Rep 2004;8:463–7.
12. Simons DG, Travell JG, Simons LS. Travell and Simon's myofascial pain and dysfunction: the trigger point manual. 2nd edition. Baltimore (MD): Williams and Wilkins; 1998.
13. Fischer AA. Pressure threshold meter: its use for quantification of tender points. Arch Phys Med Rehabil 1986;67:836.
14. Hong C-Z, Chen Y-N, Twehous D, et al. Pressure threshold for referred pain by compression on the trigger point and adjacent areas. Journal of Musculoskeletal Pain 1996;4:61–79.
15. Hubbard D, Berkhoff G. Myofascial trigger points show spontaneous needle EMG activity. Spine 1993;18:1803–7.
16. Simons DG, Hong C-Z, Simons LS. Prevalence of spontaneous electrical activity at trigger spots and at control sites in rabbit skeletal muscle. Journal of Musculoskeletal Pain 1995;3:35–48.
17. Graff-Redford SB, Reeves JL, Baker RL, et al. Effects of transcutaneous electrical nerve stimulation on myofascial pain and trigger point sensitivity. Pain 1989;37:1–5.
18. Ruane J. Identifying and injecting myofascial trigger points. Phys Sportsmed 2001;29(12):49–53.
19. Hong C-Z, Simons DG. Response to standard treatment for pectoralis minor myofascial pain syndrome after whiplash. Journal of Musculoskeletal Pain 1993;1:89–131.
20. Hong C-Z, Simons D. Pathophysiologic and electrophysiologic mechanisms of myofascial trigger points. Arch Phys Med Rehabil 1998;79:863–72.
21. Hubbard D. Chronic and recurrent muscle pain: pathophysiology and treatment, and review of pharmacologic studies. Journal of Musculoskeletal Pain 1996;4:123–43.
22. Acquandro MA, Borodic GE. Treatment of myofascial pain with botulism toxin A. Anesthesiology 1994;80:705–6.
23. Cheshire WP, Abashian SW, Mann JD. Botulism toxin in the treatment of myofascial pain syndrome. Pain 1994;59:65–9.
24. Chen J, Chung K, Hou C, et al. Inhibitory effect of dry needling on the spontaneous electrical activity recorded from myofascial trigger points of rabbit skeletal muscle. Am J Phys Med Rehabil 2001;80:729–35.

Documentation and Potential Tools in Long-Term Opioid Therapy for Pain

Howard S. Smith, MD, FACP[a],*, Kenneth L. Kirsh, PhD[b]

KEY WORDS

• Pain • Opioids • Documentation

Tremendous progress has been made in the study and treatment of pain in the past 2 decades.[1,2] Efforts have been undertaken to make pain assessment and treatment a priority of medical care and to use all of the weapons in our arsenal to bring relief to the millions of people with chronic pain.[3,4] However, this progress has been somewhat tempered by the souring of the regulatory climate and the growth of prescription drug abuse. Because of this, there has been a trend for clinicians to shy away from using high opioid doses or even using this modality at all in the treatment of chronic pain.[5–7]

Despite these setbacks, the use of long-term opioid therapy (LTOT) to treat chronic noncancer pain is growing, based in part on evidence from clinical trials and a growing consensus among pain specialists.[8–12] The appropriate use of these drugs requires skills in opioid prescribing, knowledge of addiction medicine principles, and a commitment to perform and document a comprehensive assessment repeatedly over time. Inadequate assessment can lead to undertreatment, compromise the effectiveness of therapy when implemented, and prevent an appropriate response when problematic drug-related behaviors occur.[13–15]

Fortunately, there is a growing interest in the development of tools that can be useful for screening patients up front to determine relative risk for patients having problems with prescription drug abuse or misuse. Regarding brief screening instruments, a number have arisen, including the Screening Tool for Addiction Risk (STAR),[16] Drug Abuse Screening Test (DAST),[17] Screener and Opioid Assessment for Patients with Pain (SOAPP),[18] and the Opioid Risk Tool (ORT)[19] among others. The choice in

This article originally appeared in *Medical Clinics of North America*, Volume 91, Issue 2.

[a] Albany Medical College, Department of Anesthesiology, 47 New Scotland Avenue, MC-131 Albany, NY 12208, USA

[b] Pharmacy Practice and Science, University of Kentucky, 725 Rose Street, 401C, Lexington, KY 40536-0082, USA

* Corresponding author.

E-mail address: SmithH@mail.amc.edu (H.S. Smith).

tools for more thorough ongoing assessment, however, has been somewhat more limited up until now and will be the focus of our discussion.

Regulatory agencies, state medical boards, and various peer-review groups among others not only expect appropriate medical care but also require proper documentation. In cases of LTOT for chronic pain, aside from the usual "SOAP" (ie, subjective/objective/assessment/plan)-style medical progress notes, various other issues may deserve documentation. Although there are no explicit requirements spelled out as to what and how to document issues related to LTOT, it is felt by some that the use of specific tools/instruments in the chart on some or all visits may boost adherence to documentation expectations as well as consistency of such documentation. Assessment tools may also be helpful in the analysis of persistent pain.[20]

It must be cautioned that physicians who adequately assess patients before and during opioid therapy may still encounter problems as a result of poor documentation. In a chart review of 300 patients with chronic pain, 61% had no documentation of a treatment plan.[21] Similarly, a review of the initial consultation notes of 513 patients with acute musculoskeletal pain revealed that only 43% of historical findings and 28% of physical examination findings were documented.[22] In a review of 520 randomly selected visits at an outpatient oncology practice, quantitative assessment of pain scores occurred in less than 1% of cases and qualitative assessment of pain occurred in only 60% of cases.[23] Finally, a review of medical records of 111 randomly selected patients who underwent urine toxicology screens in a cancer center found that documentation was infrequent: 37.8% of physicians failed to list a reason for the test, and 89% of the charts did not include the results of the test.[24]

AREAS OF INTEREST FOR DOCUMENTATION

Clearly, strategies are needed to translate these recommendations for patient assessment during long-term opioid therapy to frontline practice. This effort would certainly benefit from the availability of a consistent method of documentation. As one potential framework, it is important to consider four main domains in assessing pain outcomes and to better protect your practice for those patients you maintain on an opioid regimen: (1) pain relief, (2) functional outcomes, (3) side effects, and (4) drug-related behaviors. These domains have been labeled the "Four A's" (Analgesia, Activities of daily living, Adverse effects, and Aberrant drug-related behaviors) for teaching purposes.[25] There are, of course, many different ways to think about these domains, and multiple attempts to capture them will be discussed in this article.

THE PAIN ASSESSMENT AND DOCUMENTATION TOOL

The Pain Assessment and Documentation Tool (PADT) is a simple charting device based on the 4 A's concept that is designed to focus on key outcomes and provide a consistent way to document progress in pain management therapy over time. Twenty-seven clinicians completed the preliminary version of the PADT for 388 opioid-treated patients.[26,27] Nineteen clinicians (17 physicians, 1 nurse, and 1 psychologist) participated in a debriefing phase. Twelve of the 19 clinicians had participated in the field trial before the debriefing. The debriefing interview for these clinicians used the same standard questions to evaluate both the original and revised PADT.

The result of this work is a brief, two-sided chart note that can be readily included in the patient's medical record. It was designed to be intuitive, pragmatic, and adaptable to clinical situations. In the field trial, it took clinicians between 10 and 20 minutes to complete the tool. The revised PADT is substantially shorter and should require a few minutes to complete. By addressing the need for documentation, the PADT can assist clinicians in meeting their obligations for ongoing assessment and documentation. Although the PADT is not intended to replace a progress note, it is well suited to complement existing documentation with a focused evaluation of outcomes that are clinically relevant and address the need for evidence of appropriate monitoring.

The decision to assess the four domains subsumed under the shorthand designation, the "Four A's," was based on clinical experience, the positive comments received by the investigators during educational programs on opioid pharmacotherapy for noncancer pain, and an evolving national movement that recognizes the need to approach opioid therapy with a "balanced" response. This response recognizes both the legitimate need to provide optimal therapy to appropriate patients and the need to acknowledge the potential for abuse, diversion, and addiction.[25] The value of assessing pain relief, side effects, and aspects of functioning has been emphasized repeatedly in the literature.[21,28–31] Documentation of drug-related behaviors is a relatively new concept that is being explored for the first time in the PADT.

ASSESSING OPIOID THERAPY ADVERSE EFFECTS

Documentation of adverse effects in a majority of charts from many pain clinics tend to be addressed (or in many cases not addressed) in their charts by a brief note of the presence or absence of one or more adverse effects (eg, nausea, constipation, itching), noted by busy clinicians. Similar to the goal of the PADT, having a standardized form that is used at every visit and filled out by the patients before being seen by health care providers may provide certain advantages.

Patients with persistent pain on oral opioid therapy have asked to "come off" the opioids because of adverse effects, even if they perceived that opioids were providing reasonable analgesic effects.[32] The distress that may be caused by opioid adverse effects may also be seen with acute postoperative pain patients, who may occasionally ask to stop their opioids despite that they are perceived as effective analgesics, because of the significant distress and suffering that they perceive they are experiencing from an opioid adverse effect.

It therefore appears crucial to assess opioid adverse effects. Ideally, this should be done in a manner as to be able to follow trends as well as compare the patients' perceived intensity of the adverse effects versus the intensity of pain or other symptoms or adverse effects.

One available tool for the quantification of adverse effects is the Numerical Opioid Side Effect (NOSE) assessment tool (see **Fig. 1**).[33] The NOSE instrument is self-administered, can be completed by the patient in minutes, and can be entered into electronic databases or inserted into a hard-copy chart on each patient visit. The NOSE assessment tool is easy to administer as well as easy to interpret and may provide clinicians with important clinical information that could potentially impact various therapeutic decisions. Although most clinicians probably routinely assess adverse effects of treatments, it is sometimes difficult to find legible, clear, and concise documentation of such information in outpatient records. Furthermore, the documentation that does exist may not always attempt to "quantify" the intensity of treatment-related adverse effects or lend itself to looking at trends.

ASSESSING LTOT EFFICACY

The Initiative on Methods, Measurements, and Pain Assessment in Clinical Trials (IMMPACT) recommended that six core outcome domains ([1]pain, [2]physical functions, [3]emotion, [4]participant rating of improvement and satisfaction with treatment,

	Not Present									As Bad As You Can Imagine	
	0	1	2	3	4	5	6	7	8	9	10
1. Nausea, vomiting, and/or lack of appetite	O	O	O	O	O	O	O	O	O	O	O
2. Fatigue, sleepiness, trouble concentrating, hallucinations, and/or drowsiness/somnolence	O	O	O	O	O	O	O	O	O	O	O
3. Constipation	O	O	O	O	O	O	O	O	O	O	O
4. Itching	O	O	O	O	O	O	O	O	O	O	O
5. Decreased sexual desire/function and/or diminished libido	O	O	O	O	O	O	O	O	O	O	O
6. Dry Mouth	O	O	O	O	O	O	O	O	O	O	O
7. Abdominal pain or discomfort/cramping or bloating	O	O	O	O	O	O	O	O	O	O	O
8. Sweating	O	O	O	O	O	O	O	O	O	O	O
9. Headache and/or dizziness	O	O	O	O	O	O	O	O	O	O	O
10. Urinary retention	O	O	O	O	O	O	O	O	O	O	O

Fig. 1. Numerical Opioid Side Effect (NOSE) assessment tool.

[5]symptoms and adverse events, and [6]participant disposition) should be considered when designing chronic pain clinical trials.[34] The authors believe that the use of a unidimensional tool such as the numerical rating scale-11 (NRS-11) provides a suboptimal assessment of chronic pain as well as LTOT efficacy. Clinicians should attempt to assess multiple domains (preferably with multidimensional tools) in efforts to achieve a global picture of the patient's baseline status as well as the patient's response to LTOT in various domains.

It has been proposed that the use of a collection of various tools may provide adjunct information and help clinicians to create a more complete picture regarding longitudinal trends of overall progress/functioning for their patients with chronic pain on LTOT.[35] Assessing individual outcomes during outpatient multidisciplinary chronic pain treatment is often an extremely challenging task. There are many tools and instruments currently available, but the Treatment Outcomes in Pain Survey tool (TOPS) has been specifically designed to assess and follow outcomes in the chronic pain population and has been described as an augmented SF-36.[36,37] The Medical Outcomes Study (MOS) Short Form 36-item questionnaire (SF-36) compares the health status of large populations without a preponderance of one single medical condition.[38] The SF-36 assesses eight domains, but it has not been found to be especially useful for following the changes in function and pain in chronic pain populations.

The eight domains of the SF-36 are bodily pain (BP), general health (GH), mental health (MH), physical functioning (PF), role emotional (RE), social functioning (SF), role physical (RP), and vitality (VT). The TOPS scale initially had nine domains, but one (satisfaction with outcomes) was modified in subsequent versions. The nine domains of TOPS are Pain Symptom, Family/Social Disability, Functional Limitations,

Total Pain Experience, Objective Work Disability, Life Control, Solicitous Responses, Passive Coping, and Satisfaction with Outcomes. This enhanced SF-36 (TOPS scale) was constructed by obtaining patient data from the SF-36 with 12 additional role-functioning questions. These additional questions were taken in part from the 61-item Multidimensional Pain Inventory (MPI)[39] and the 10-item Oswestry Disability Questionnaire,[40] with four additional pain-related questions that are similar to those found in the MOS pain-related questions,[41] the Brief Pain Inventory,[28] and a six-item coping scale from the MOS.[41]

The question adapted from the Oswestry Disability Questionnaire (designed for back pain patients) includes questions that relate to impairment (pain), physical functioning (how long the patient can sit or stand), and disability (ability to travel or have sexual relations).[40] The patient-generated index is an instrument that attempts to individualize a patient's perception of his or her quality of life.[42]

Although the TOPS instrument is an extremely useful tool, it is time-consuming, is based entirely on the patient's subjective responses, and requires that the clinician has access, whether by a special computer program or by sending forms away, for scoring. As a result, it may not be an ideal instrument to use in every pain clinic and may not provide the clinician with an answer immediately of how the patient is doing relative to previous visits (although it may have that potential with adequate time, scanning equipment, and computer software).

TRANSLATIONAL ANALGESIA

A concept that may possess potential utility for clinicians is translational analgesia. Translational analgesia refers to improvements in physical, social, or emotional function that are realized by the patient as a result of improved analgesia, or essentially what did the pain relief experienced by the patient "translate" into in terms of perceived improved quality of life.[43] In most cases, a sustained and significant improvement in pain perception that is deemed worthwhile to the patient should "translate" into improvement in quality of life or improved social, emotional, or physical function. Improvements in social, emotional, or physical domains are often spontaneously reported by patients, but in most cases should be able to be ascertained or elicited via "focused" interview techniques with the patient, significant others, and family; "focused" physical exam; or a combination of any of these. Improvements may be subtle and could include a range of daily function activities or other signs (eg, going out more with friends, doing laundry, showing improved mood/relations with family members). It is important to note that this issue is certainly not exclusive to opioid therapy and is thought to apply to other treatments.

The authors do not deem it inappropriate or inhumane to taper relatively "high-dose" opioid therapy in a patient with chronic pain who notes that his or her NRS-11 "pain score" has dropped from 9/10 to 8/10 after escalating to over a gram of long-acting morphine preparation per day but in whom the patient as well as the patient's family or significant other cannot describe (and the clinician cannot elicit) any significant "translational analgesia." A patient with chronic pain who demonstrates a failure to "get off the couch," despite equivocal or minimally improved analgesia, should not be considered as a therapeutic success. But, should this viewpoint be seen as cruel or as a punishment for these patients? Rome and colleagues[44] demonstrated that at least a subpopulation of patients seems to do better after tapering off opioids. Furthermore, more evidence regarding the hyperalgesic actions of opioids in certain circumstances is mounting.[45,46]

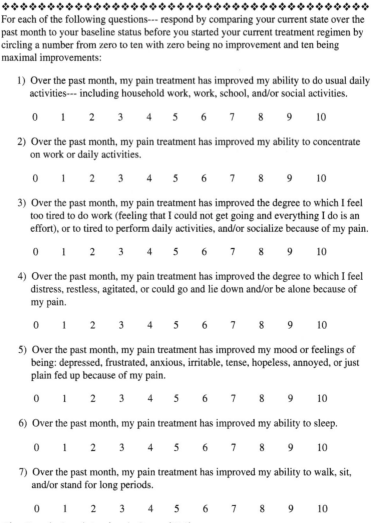

❖❖

For each of the following questions--- respond by comparing your current state over the past month to your baseline status before you started your current treatment regimen by circling a number from zero to ten with zero being no improvement and ten being maximal improvements:

1) Over the past month, my pain treatment has improved my ability to do usual daily activities--- including household work, work, school, and/or social activities.

   0   1   2   3   4   5   6   7   8   9   10

2) Over the past month, my pain treatment has improved my ability to concentrate on work or daily activities.

   0   1   2   3   4   5   6   7   8   9   10

3) Over the past month, my pain treatment has improved the degree to which I feel too tired to do work (feeling that I could not get going and everything I do is an effort), or to tired to perform daily activities, and/or socialize because of my pain.

   0   1   2   3   4   5   6   7   8   9   10

4) Over the past month, my pain treatment has improved the degree to which I feel distress, restless, agitated, or could go and lie down and/or be alone because of my pain.

   0   1   2   3   4   5   6   7   8   9   10

5) Over the past month, my pain treatment has improved my mood or feelings of being: depressed, frustrated, anxious, irritable, tense, hopeless, annoyed, or just plain fed up because of my pain.

   0   1   2   3   4   5   6   7   8   9   10

6) Over the past month, my pain treatment has improved my ability to sleep.

   0   1   2   3   4   5   6   7   8   9   10

7) Over the past month, my pain treatment has improved my ability to walk, sit, and/or stand for long periods.

   0   1   2   3   4   5   6   7   8   9   10

Fig. 2. The Translational Analgesic Score (TAS).

The periodic assessment of the patient with chronic pain should be performed in multiple domains (eg, social domain, analgesia domain, functional domain, emotional domain). The authors believe the relatively common practice of evaluating patients with chronic pain by obtaining an NRS-11 pain score at each assessment and basing opioid analgesic treatment solely on this score to be suboptimal. Although tools exist that assess multiple domains used in research, there is no simple, convenient, and universally acceptable instrument that is used in busy clinical pain practices.

To address this issue, a recent tool has been developed. The SAFE score (see section titled "The SAFE score") is a multidomain assessment tool that may have potential utility for rapid dynamic assessment in the busy clinic setting.[47,48] The SAFE score is a clinician-generated tool and may best be used in conjunction with the translational analgesic score (TAS) (a patient-generated tool) as an adjunct. These are discussed, in turn, in the following two sections.

8) Over the past month, my pain treatment has improved my ability to go up stairs, and/or move or lift objects.

0   1   2   3   4   5   6   7   8   9   10

9) Over the past month, my pain treatment has improved the extent to which my pain interferes with optimal interpersonal relationships and/or intimacy.

0   1   2   3   4   5   6   7   8   9   10

10) Over the past month, to what degree have you, your significant other, your family, your co-workers, and/or your friends noticed any improvements in your socializing, recreational activities, physical functioning, concentration, mood, interpersonal relationships, activities of daily living, and/or overall quality of life?

0   1   2   3   4   5   6   7   8   9   10

--- Please write below--- specific examples of things you can now do or currently do frequently that you couldn't do or only did rarely when your pain was not controlled as well as it is now.

<u>**TAS**</u> = _____

❖❖❖

The TAS is expressed as a number between 0 to 10 with a decimal being the average of the responses to the ten questions (or less--- if the patient is paraplegic then they would not answer the questions regarding going up stairs, etc.).

As an example, a patient's response to the TAS tool is shown below:
   1) Over the past month, my pain treatment has improved my ability to do usual daily activities--- including household work, work, school, and/or social activities.

0   1   2   3   •   5   6   7   8   9   10

   2) Over the past month, my pain treatment has improved my ability to concentrate on work or daily activities.

0   1   2   •   4   5   6   7   8   9   10

   3) Over the past month, my pain treatment has improved the degree to which I feel too tired to do work (feeling that I could not get going and everything I do is an effort), or to tired to perform daily activities, and/or socialize because of my pain.

0   1   2   •   4   5   6   7   8   9   10

Fig. 2. (continued)

THE TRANSLATIONAL ANALGESIC SCORE

The translational analgesic score (TAS) is a patient-generated tool that attempts to quantify the degree of "translational analgesia" (see **Fig. 2**).[48] It is simple, rapid, user-friendly, and suitable for use in busy pain clinics. The patient can be handed the TAS sheet with questions to fill out at each visit while in the waiting room and the responses are averaged for an overall score that is recorded in the chart. The authors encourage clinicians to have all patients write down specific examples of things that they can now do or do frequently that they couldn't do or did rarely

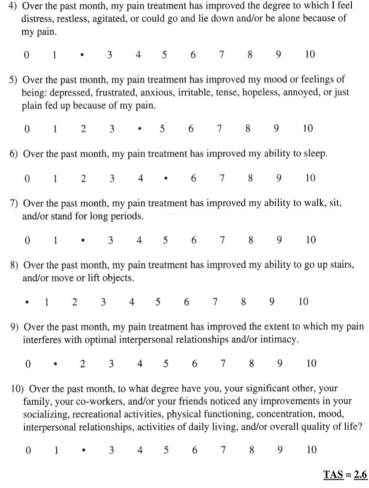

4) Over the past month, my pain treatment has improved the degree to which I feel distress, restless, agitated, or could go and lie down and/or be alone because of my pain.

0   1   •   3   4   5   6   7   8   9   10

5) Over the past month, my pain treatment has improved my mood or feelings of being: depressed, frustrated, anxious, irritable, tense, hopeless, annoyed, or just plain fed up because of my pain.

0   1   2   3   •   5   6   7   8   9   10

6) Over the past month, my pain treatment has improved my ability to sleep.

0   1   2   3   4   •   6   7   8   9   10

7) Over the past month, my pain treatment has improved my ability to walk, sit, and/or stand for long periods.

0   1   •   3   4   5   6   7   8   9   10

8) Over the past month, my pain treatment has improved my ability to go up stairs, and/or move or lift objects.

•   1   2   3   4   5   6   7   8   9   10

9) Over the past month, my pain treatment has improved the extent to which my pain interferes with optimal interpersonal relationships and/or intimacy.

0   •   2   3   4   5   6   7   8   9   10

10) Over the past month, to what degree have you, your significant other, your family, your co-workers, and/or your friends noticed any improvements in your socializing, recreational activities, physical functioning, concentration, mood, interpersonal relationships, activities of daily living, and/or overall quality of life?

0   1   •   3   4   5   6   7   8   9   10

TAS = 2.6

Fig. 2. (continued)

when their pain was less controlled. Alternatively, the patients' responses can be entered into a computerized record (with graphs of trends) if the pain clinic's medical records are electronic.

In the sample provided, the patient answered all 10 questions with responses, hence, the average is the sum of all responses (26) divided by 10. Therefore, the TAS is 2.6. A patient, who at each visit consistently has a TAS of 10.0, clearly represents a therapeutic success on their current treatment. Conversely, a patient who at each visit consistently has a TAS of 0.0 would represent a suboptimal therapeutic result (by TAS criteria). Clinicians are encouraged to document at least one or two specific examples of translational analgesia (eg, perhaps various activities that the patient can now perform as a result of pain relief or can now perform frequently as a result of pain relief that the patient could not do or only do infrequently before therapy) on the bottom or reverse side of the TAS score sheet. Treatment decisions regarding escalation or tapering of opioids, changing agents, adding agents, obtaining consultations, instituting physical medicine or behavioral medicine techniques, remain

	Rating	Criterion				
Social Marital, family, friends, leisure, recreational		1 supportive harmonious socializing engaged	2	3	4	5 conflictual discord isolated bored
Analgesia Intensity, frequency, duration		1 comfortable effective controlled	2	3	4	5 intolerable ineffective uncontrolled
Function Work, ADL's, home management, school, training, physical activity		1 independent active productive energetic	2	3	4	5 dependent unmotivated passive deconditioned
Emotional Cognitive, stress, attitude, mood, behavior, neuro- vegetative signs		1 clear relaxed optimistic upbeat composed	2	3	4	5 confused tense pessimistic depressed distressed
Total Score						

The patient's status in each of the four domains is rated as follows:

1 = Excellent
2 = Good
3 = Fair
4 = Borderline
5 = Poor

Fig. 3. Sample SAFE form.

the medical judgment of practitioners and should be based on a careful reevaluation of the patient and not based on a number.

The concept of translational analgesia is not meant to imply that opioids should be tapered, weaned, or discontinued. If a patient has a TAS that is very low and essentially unchanged over time (especially in conjunction with a SAFE score in the "red zone"), then this should prompt the clinician to reevaluate the patient and consider a change in therapy. This could mean pursuing various therapeutic options including perhaps increasing the dose of opioids. However, if a patient has a high TAS and a SAFE score in the green zone, the patient should probably continue LTOT.

THE SAFE SCORE

Another tool that has been advocated to help with this purpose is called the SAFE score.[47,48] Although it has not yet been rigorously validated, it is simple and practical and may possess clinical utility. It is a score generated by the health care provider that

Example A

Social	3
Analgesia	2
Function	3
Emotional	3
Green Zone "SAFE" score	11

Example B

Social	2
Analgesia	4
Function	3
Emotional	1
Green Zone "SAFE" score	10

Fig. 4. Green zone cases using the SAFE scoring tool.

Example C

Social	5
Analgesia	3
Function	5
Emotional	5
Red Zone "SAFE" score	18

Example D

Social	3
Analgesia	4
Function	3
Emotional	3
Green Zone "SAFE" score	13

Fig. 5. Tracking an overall positive change in status using the SAFE scoring tool.

is meant to reflect a multidimensional assessment of outcome to opioid therapy. It is not meant to replace more elaborate patient-based assessment tools but could possibly serve as an adjunct and possibly in the future shed some light on the difference between patients' perception of how they are doing on opioid treatment versus the physician-based view of outcome.

At each visit, the clinician rates the patient's functioning and pain relief in four domains. The domains assessed include social functioning (S), analgesia or pain relief (A), physical functioning (F), and emotional functioning (E). Together, the ratings in each of the four domains are combined to yield a "SAFE" score. The "SAFE" score can range from 4 to 20.

The SAFE tool is both practical in its ease and clinically useful (**Fig. 3**). The goals of the SAFE tool are multifold. Specifically, they include the need to demonstrate that the clinician has routinely evaluated the efficacy of the treatment from multiple perspectives; guide the clinician toward a broader view of treatment options beyond adjusting the medication regimen; and document the clinician's rationale for continuation, modification, or cessation of opioid therapy.

INTERPRETATION OF SCORES

Scores can be broken down into three distinct categories. First, the *green zone* represents a SAFE score of 4 to 12 or decrease of 2 points in total score from baseline. With a score in the green zone, the patient is considered to be doing well and the plan would be to continue with the current medication regimen or consider reducing the total dose of the opioids. Second, the *yellow zone* represents a SAFE score of 13 to 16 or a rating of 5 in any category or an increase of 2 or more from baseline in the total score. With a score in the yellow zone, the patient should be monitored closely and reassessed frequently. Finally, the *red zone* represents a SAFE score greater than or equal to 17. With a score in the red zone, a change in the treatment would be warranted.

Once the color determination is made, a decision can be made regarding treatment options. Treatment options depend on the pattern of scores. If attempts are made to address problems in specific domains and the patient is still not showing an

Example E

Social	3
Analgesia	2
Function	3
Emotional	3
Green Zone "SAFE" score	11

Example F

Social	3
Analgesia	2
Function	4
Emotional	4
Yellow Zone "SAFE" score	13

Fig. 6. Tracking an overall negative change in status using the SAFE scoring tool.

improvement in the SAFE score, then the patient may not be an appropriate candidate for long-term opioid therapy.

Fig. 4 illustrates green zone cases. In example A, there is good analgesic response to opioids, with a fair response in the other domains. No change in treatment would be necessary unless adverse reactions to the medications require an adjustment or discontinuation. In example B, there is borderline analgesic response, but good social and emotional responses and a fair physical functioning response. Some pain specialists may determine that the medication regimen should be optimized. For others, this pattern of ratings may reflect a reasonable improvement in quality of life for the patient. Therefore, continuing the present medication regimen would be a reasonable option.

Fig. 5 illustrates how the SAFE tool can be used to track changes in the status of the same patient on two consecutive visits. In the change in scores from example C to example D, although analgesia deteriorates from fair to borderline, there is significant improvement in the other domains. The clinician may feel this is satisfactory for this particular patient and continue with the current medication regimen. Once again, too narrow a focus on analgesic response may lead to unnecessary dose escalation. This case also illustrates the situation in which even though the total score at visit D is greater than 12 and would be a *yellow zone*, it is assigned as a *green zone* because there was a decrease of more than 2 in the total score. Alternately, the clinician may determine that a borderline analgesic response is not optimal. The choices for intervention may include rotating to another opioid agent, increasing the current opioid dose, adding adjuvant medications, referring for nonpharmacological treatment, or discontinuing high-dose opioids.

Fig. 6 illustrates again a single patient on two consecutive visits. Here, analgesia has remained good over time, but there has been a negative impact on the domains of function and emotion. Pain specialists who are focused on the pain scores of such a patient may be comfortable with continuing the established treatment plan. However, using SAFE, an expanded view of the patient's overall status will alert the clinician to monitor the patient's physical and emotional functioning in future visits. If the ratings in the psychological and physical domains persist, then the clinician may recommend that the patient pursue psychosocial treatment or physical rehabilitation in addition to maintaining the medication regimen.

SUMMARY

Assessment and documentation are cornerstones for both protecting your practice and obtaining optimal patient outcomes while on opioid therapy. There are a growing number of assessment tools for clinicians to guide the evaluation of a group of important outcomes during opioid therapy and provide a simple means of documenting patient care. They all have the capability to prove helpful in clinical management and offer mechanisms for documenting the types of practice standards that those in the regulatory and law enforcement communities seek to ensure.

REFERENCES

1. Berry PH, Dahl JL. The new JCAHO pain standards: implications for pain management nurses. Pain Manag Nurs 2000;1(1):3–12.
2. SUPPORT Study Principal Investigators. A controlled trial to improve care for seriously ill hospitalized patients: a study to understand prognoses and preferences for outcomes and risks of treatment (SUPPORT). JAMA 1995;274:1591.
3. Osterweis M, Kleinman A, Mechanic D, editors. Pain and disability: clinical, behavioral, and public policy perspectives. [Report of the Committee on Pain,

Disability, and Chronic Illness Behavior, Institute of Medicine, National Academy of Sciences.]. Washington, DC: National Academy Press; 1987.

4. Verhaak PFM, Kerssens JJ, Dekker J, et al. Prevalence of chronic benign pain disorder among adults: a review of the literature. Pain 1998;77:231–9.

5. Cicero TJ, Inciardi JA, Munoz A. Trends in abuse of Oxycontin and other opioid analgesics in the United States: 2002–2004. J Pain 2005;6(10):662–72.

6. Lipman AG. Does the DEA truly seek balance in pain medicine? J Pain Palliat Care Pharmacother 2005;19(1):7–9.

7. Passik SD, Kirsh KL. Fear and loathing in the pain clinic. Pain Med 2006;7(4): 363–4.

8. Collett BJ. Opioid tolerance: the clinical perspective. Br J Anaesth 1998;81: 58–68.

9. Portenoy RK. Opioid therapy for chronic nonmalignant pain: a review of critical issues. J Pain Symptom Manage 1996;11:203–17.

10. Portenoy RK. Opioid therapy for chronic nonmalignant pain. Pain Res Manage 1996;1:17–28.

11. Urban BJ, France RD, Steinberger EK, et al. Long-term use of narcotic/antidepressant medication in the management of phantom limb pain. Pain 1986;24: 191–6.

12. Zenz M, Strumpf M, Tryba M. Long-term oral opioid therapy in patients with chronic nonmalignant pain. J Pain Symptom Manage 1992;7:69–77.

13. Joint Commission on the Accreditation of Healthcare Organizations. Patient rights and organization ethics. Referenced from the comprehensive accreditation manual for hospitals, update 3, 1999. Available at: http://www.jointcommission. org. Accessed September 2006.

14. Max MB, Payne R, Edwards WT, et al. Principles of analgesic use in the treatment of acute pain and cancer pain. 4th edition. Glenview, IL: American Pain Society; 1999.

15. Katz N. The impact of pain management on quality of life. J Pain Symptom Manage 2002;24(suppl 1):S38–47.

16. Friedman R, Li V, Mehrotra D. Treating pain patients at risk: evaluation of a screening tool in opioid-treated pain patients with and without addiction. Pain Med 2003;4(2):182–5.

17. Gavin DR, Ross HE, Skinner HA. Diagnostic validity of the drug abuse screening test in the assessment of DSM-III drug disorders. Br J Addict 1989;84(3):301–7.

18. Butler SF, Budman SH, Fernandez K, et al. Validation of a screener and opioid assessment measure for patients with chronic pain. Pain 2004;112(1–2):65–75.

19. Webster LR, Webster RM. Predicting aberrant behaviors in opioid-treated patients: preliminary validation of the Opioid Risk Tool. Pain Med 2005;6(6): 432–42.

20. Wincent A, Linden Y, Arner S. Pain questionnaires in the analysis of long lasting (chronic) pain conditions. Eur J Pain 2003;7:311–21.

21. Clark JD. Chronic pain prevalence and analgesic prescribing in a general medical population. J Pain Symptom Manage 2002;23:131–7.

22. Solomon DH, Schaffer JL, Katz JN, et al. Can history and physical examination be used as markers of quality? An analysis of the initial visit note in musculoskeletal care. Med Care 2000;38:383–91.

23. Rhodes DJ, Koshy RC, Waterfield WC, et al. Feasibility of quantitative pain assessment in outpatient oncology practice. J Clin Oncol 2001;19:501–8.

24. Passik SD, Schreiber J, Kirsh KL, et al. A chart review of the ordering and documentation of urine toxicology screens in a cancer center: do they influence patient management? J Pain Symptom Manage 2000;19:40–4.

25. Passik SD, Weinreb HJ. Managing chronic nonmalignant pain: overcoming obstacles to the use of opioids. Adv Ther 2000;17:70–83.
26. Passik SD, Kirsh KL, Whitcomb LA, et al. A new tool to assess and document pain outcomes in chronic pain patients receiving opioid therapy. Clin Ther 2004;26(4): 552–61.
27. Passik SD, Kirsh KL, Whitcomb LA, et al. Monitoring outcomes during long-term opioid therapy for non-cancer pain: results with the pain assessment and documentation tool. Journal of Opioid Management 2005;1(5):257–66.
28. Daut R, Cleeland C, Flannery R. Development of the Wisconsin Brief Pain Questionnaire to assess pain in cancer and other diseases. Pain 1983;17: 197–210.
29. Cleeland CS, Ryan KM. Pain assessment: global use of the Brief Pain Inventory. Ann Acad Med Singapore 1994;23:129–38.
30. Melzack R. The McGill Pain Questionnaire: major properties and scoring methods. Pain 1975;1:277–99.
31. McCarberg BH, Barkin RL. Long-acting opioids for chronic pain: pharmacotherapeutic opportunities to enhance compliance, quality of life, and analgesia. Am J Ther 2001;8:181–6.
32. Kalso E, Edwards JE, Moore RA, et al. Opioids in chronic non-cancer pain: systematic review of efficacy and safety. Pain 2004;112:372–80.
33. Smith HS. The Numerical Opioid Side Effect (NOSE). Assessment tool. Journal of Cancer Pain and Symptom Palliation 2005;1:3–6.
34. Turk DC, Dworkin RH, Allen RR, et al. Core outcome domains for chronic pain clinical trials: IMMPACT recommendations. Pain 2003;106:337–45.
35. Smith HS. Translational analgesia and the translational analgesic score. Journal of Cancer Pain and Symptom Palliation 2005;1:15–9.
36. Rogers WH, Wittink H, Wagner A, et al. Assessing individual outcomes during outpatient multidisciplinary chronic pain treatment by means of an augmented SF-36. Pain Med 2000;1:44–54.
37. Rogers WH, Wittink H, Ashburn MA, et al. Using the "TOPS," an outcome instrument for multidisciplinary outpatient pain treatment. Pain Med 2000;1:55–67.
38. Ware JE Jr, Sherbourne CD, The MOS. 36-item short-form health survey (SF-36). I. Conceptual Framework and Item Selection. Med Care 1992;30:473–83.
39. Kerns R, Turk D, Rudy T. The West Haven-Yale Multidimensional Pain Inventory (WHYMPI). Pain 1985;23:345–6.
40. Fairbanks J, Couper J, Davies J, et al. The Oswestry low back pain disability questionnaire. Physiotherapy 1980;66:271–3.
41. Tarlor A, Ware J Jr, Greenfield S, et al. The Medical Outcomes Study: an application of methods for monitoring the results of medical care. JAMA 1989;262: 925–30.
42. Ruta DA, Garratt AM, Leng M, et al. A new approach to quality of life: the patient-generated index. Med Care 1994;32:1109–26.
43. Smith HS. Perspectives in persistent noncancer pain. Journal of Cancer Pain and Symptom Palliation 2005c;1:31–2.
44. Rome JD, Townsend CP, Bruce BK, et al. Chronic noncancer pain rehabilitation with opioid withdrawal: comparison of treatment outcomes based on opioid use status at admission. Mayo Clin Proc 2004;79:759–68.
45. Holtman JR, Wala EP. Characterization of morphine-induced hyperalgesia in male and female rats. Pain 2005;114:62–70.
46. Ruscheweyh R, Sand Kuhler J. Opioids and central sensitization: II. Induction and reversal of hyperalgesia. Eur J Pain 2005;9:149–52.

47. Smith H, Audette J, Witkower A. Assessing analgesic therapeutic outcomes. In: Smith H, editor. Drugs for pain. Philadelphia (PA): H. Hanley and Belfus; 2003. p. 499–508.
48. Smith HS, Audette J, Witkower A. Playing It "SAFE". Journal of Cancer Pain and Symptom Palliation 2005;1:3–10.

Nonopioid Analgesics

Muhammad A. Munir, MD*, Nasr Enany, MD,
Jun-Ming Zhang, MSc, MD

KEYWORDS

• Pain • Analgesics • Nonopioids • Coanalgesics • NSAIDs

Drug therapy is the mainstay of management for acute, chronic, and cancer pain in all age groups, including neonates, infants, and children. The analgesics include opioids, nonopioid analgesics, and adjuvants or coanalgesics. In this article we will overview various nonopioid analgesics including salicylates, acetaminophen, traditional nonselective nonsteroidal anti-inflammatory drugs (NSAIDs), and cyclooxygenase-2 (COX-2) inhibitors. Unless contraindicated, any analgesic regimen should include a nonopioid drug, even when pain is severe enough to require the addition of an opioid.[1]

NONOPIOID ANALGESICS

Acetaminophen and NSAIDs are useful for acute and chronic pain resulting from a variety of disease processes including trauma, arthritis, surgery, and cancer.[2,3] NSAIDs are indicated for pain that involves inflammation as an underlying pathologic process because of their ability to suppress production of inflammatory prostaglandins. NSAIDs are both analgesic and anti-inflammatory, and may be useful for the treatment of pain not involving inflammation as well.[4]

Nonopioid analgesics differ from opioid analgesics in certain important regards. These differences should be realized to provide the most effective care to acute pain patients and include the following:

1. There is a ceiling effect to the dose response curve of NSAIDs, therefore after achieving an analgesic ceiling, increasing the dose increases the side effects but additional analgesia does not result.
2. NSAIDs don't produce physical or psychological dependence and therefore sudden interruption in treatment doesn't cause drug withdrawals.
3. NSAIDs are antipyretic.

This article originally appeared in *Medical Clinics of North America*, Volume 91, Issue 1.
This work was partly supported by Grant No. NS45594 from the National Institutes of Health.
Department of Anesthesiology, University of Cincinnati College of Medicine, 231 Albert Sabin Way, PO Box 67031, Cincinnati, OH 45267-0531, USA
* Corresponding author.
E-mail address: munirma@ucmail.uc.edu (M.A. Munir).

Nonopioid analgesics are underrated for the treatment of chronic pain and unnecessarily omitted for patients with chronic pain and patients unable to take oral medications. Parenteral, topical, and rectal dosage forms are available for some NSAIDs that are often underused.

All NSAIDs, including the subclass of selective COX-2 inhibitors, are anti-inflammatory, analgesic, and antipyretic. NSAIDs are a chemically heterogeneous group of compounds, often chemically unrelated, which nevertheless share certain therapeutic actions and adverse effects. Aspirin also inhibits the COX enzymes but in a manner molecularly distinct from the competitive, reversible, active site inhibitors and is often distinguished from the NSAIDs. Similarly, acetaminophen, which is antipyretic and analgesic but largely devoid of anti-inflammatory activity, also is conventionally segregated from the group despite its sharing NSAID activity with other actions relevant to its clinical action in vivo.

MECHANISM OF ACTION

All NSAIDs inhibit the enzyme cyclooxygenase (COX), thereby inhibiting prostaglandin synthesis.[5] In addition to peripheral effects, NSAIDs exert a central action at the brain or spinal cord level that could be important for their analgesic effects.[6] More than 30 years ago, multiple isoforms of COX were hypothesized. In 1990s, the second form (COX-2) was isolated. COX-1, the originally identified isoform, is found in platelets, the gastrointestinal (GI) tract, kidneys, and most other human tissues. COX-2 is found predominantly in the kidneys and central nervous system (CNS), and is induced in peripheral tissues by noxious stimuli that cause inflammation and pain. The inhibition of COX-1 is associated with the well-known gastrointestinal bleeding and renal side effects that can occur with NSAID use. The anti-inflammatory therapeutic effects of NSAIDs are largely due to COX-2 and not the COX-1 inhibition. Until recently all available NSAIDs nonselectively inhibited the COX-1 and COX-2 isoforms. Drugs that do so are termed nonselective or traditional NSAIDs. Most NSAIDs inhibit both COX-1 and COX-2 with little selectivity, although some conventionally thought of as nonselective NSAIDs, diclofenac, etodolac, meloxicam, and nimesulide, exhibit selectivity for COX-2 in vitro. Indeed, meloxicam acts as a preferential inhibitor of COX-2 at relatively low doses (eg, 7.5 mg daily).

COX-2 selective NSAIDs that first became available in the late 1990s provide all of the beneficial effects of nonselective NSAIDs but fewer adverse effects on bleeding and the GI tract. COX-2 selective NSAIDs are no safer to the kidneys than nonselective NSAIDs. As of mid-2003, three members of the initial class of COX-2 inhibitors, the coxibs, were approved for use in the United States and Europe. Both rofecoxib and valdecoxib have now been withdrawn from the market in view of their potential cardiovascular adverse event profile. None of the coxibs have established greater clinical efficacy over NSAIDs.

Aspirin covalently modifies COX-1 and COX-2, irreversibly inhibiting cyclooxygenase activity. This is an important distinction from all the NSAIDs because the duration of aspirin's effects is related to the turnover rate of cyclooxygenases in different target tissues. The duration of effect of nonaspirin NSAIDs, which competitively inhibit the active sites of the COX enzymes, relates more directly to the time course of drug disposition. The importance of enzyme turnover in relief from aspirin action is most notable in platelets, which, being anucleate, have a markedly limited capacity for protein synthesis. Thus, the consequences of inhibition of platelet COX-1 last for the lifetime of the platelet. Inhibition of platelet COX-1-dependent thromboxane (TX)A2 formation therefore is cumulative with repeated doses of aspirin (at least as low as 30 mg/d) and takes roughly 8 to 12 days, the platelet turnover time, to recover once therapy has been stopped.

Acetaminophen is a nonsalicylate that may produce similar analgesic and antipyretic potency as aspirin, but has no antiplatelet effects, lacks clinically useful peripheral anti-inflammatory effects, and does not damage the gastric mucosa. A proposed mechanism of acetaminophen is inhibition of a third isoform of cyclooxygenase (COX-3) that was identified recently.[7] COX-3 is only found within the CNS, which would account for the analgesic and antipyretic, but not anti-inflammatory, action of acetaminophen. However, the significance of COX-3 remains uncertain, and the mechanism(s) of action of acetaminophen has yet to be defined.

Clinical Uses

All NSAIDs, including selective COX-2 inhibitors, are antipyretic, analgesic, and anti-inflammatory, with the exception of acetaminophen, which is antipyretic and analgesic but is largely devoid of anti-inflammatory activity.

Analgesic

When employed as analgesics, these drugs usually are effective only against pain of low-to-moderate intensity, such as dental pain. Although their maximal efficacy is generally much less than the opioids, NSAIDs lack the unwanted adverse effects of opiates in the CNS, including respiratory depression and the development of physical dependence. NSAIDs do not change the perception of sensory modalities other than pain. Chronic postoperative pain or pain arising from inflammation (eg, somatic pain) is controlled particularly well by NSAIDs.

Antipyretics

NSAIDs reduce fever in most situations, but not the circadian variation in temperature or the rise in response to exercise or increased ambient temperature. It is important to select an NSAID with rapid onset for the management of fever associated with minor illness in adults. Due to the association with Reye's syndrome, aspirin and other salicylates are contraindicated in children and young adults less than 12 years old with fever associated with viral illness.

Anti-inflammatory

NSAIDs have their key application as anti-inflammatory agents in the treatment of musculoskeletal disorders, such as rheumatoid arthritis and osteoarthritis. In general, NSAIDs provide only symptomatic relief from pain and inflammation associated with the disease, and do not arrest the progression of pathological injury to tissue.

OTHER CLINICAL USES

In addition to analgesic, antipyretic and anti-inflammatory effects, NSAIDs are also used for closure of patent ductus arteriosus in neonates, to treat severe episodes of vasodilatation and hypotension in systemic mastocytosis, treatment of biochemical derangement of Bartter's syndrome, chemoprevention of certain cancers such as colon cancer, and prevention of flushing associated with use of niacin.

ADVERSE REACTIONS OF NSAID TREATMENT

Adverse effects of aspirin and NSAIDs therapy are listed in **Table 1** and are considerably common in elderly patients and caution is warranted in choosing an NSAID for pain management in the elderly.

Table 1
Side effects of NSAID therapy

Gastrointestinal	Nausea, anorexia, abdominal pain, ulcers, anemia, gastrointestinal hemorrhage, perforation, diarrhea
Cardiovascular	Hypertension, decreased effectiveness of anti-hypertensive medications, myocardial infarction, stroke, and thromboembolic events (last three with selective COX-2 inhibitors); inhibit platelet activation, propensity for bruising and hemorrhage
Renal	Salt and water retention, edema, deterioration of kidney function, decreased effectiveness of diuretic medication, decreased urate excretion, hyperkalemia, analgesic nephropathy
Central nervous system	Headache, dizziness, vertigo, confusion, depression, lowering of seizure threshold, hyperventilation (salicylates)
Hypersensitivity	Vasomotor rhinitis, asthma, urticaria, flushing, hypotension, shock

Gastrointestinal

The most common symptoms associated with these drugs are gastrointestinal, including anorexia, nausea, dyspepsia, abdominal pain, and diarrhea. These symptoms may be related to the induction of gastric or intestinal ulcers, which is estimated to occur in 15% to 30% of regular users. The risk is further increased in those with *Helicobacter pylori* infection, heavy alcohol consumption, or other risk factors for mucosal injury, including the concurrent use of glucocorticoids. All of the selective COX-2 inhibitors have been shown to be less prone than equally efficacious doses of traditional NSAIDs to induce endoscopically visualized gastric ulcers.[8]

Gastric damage by NSAIDs can be brought about by at least two distinct mechanisms. Inhibition of COX-1 in gastric epithelial cells depresses mucosal cytoprotective prostaglandins, especially PGI_2 and PGE_2. These eicosanoids inhibit acid secretion by the stomach, enhance mucosal blood flow, and promote the secretion of cytoprotective mucus in the intestine. Another mechanism by which NSAIDs or aspirin may cause ulceration is by local irritation from contact of orally administered drug with the gastric mucosa.

Co-administration of the PGE_1 analog, misoprostol, or proton pump inhibitors (PPIs) in conjunction with NSAIDs can be beneficial in the prevention of duodenal and gastric ulceration.[9]

Cardiovascular

Selective inhibitors of COX-2 depress PGI_2 formation by endothelial cells without concomitant inhibition of platelet thromboxane. Experiments in mice suggest that PGI_2 restrains the cardiovascular effects of TXA_2, affording a mechanism by which selective inhibitors might increase the risk of thrombosis.[10,11] This mechanism should pertain to individuals otherwise at risk of thrombosis, such as those with rheumatoid arthritis, as the relative risk of myocardial infarction is increased in these patients compared with patients with osteoarthritis or no arthritis. The incidence of myocardial infarction and stroke has diverged in such at-risk patients when COX-2 inhibitors are compared with traditional NSAIDs.[12] Placebo-controlled trials have now revealed that there may be an increased incidence of myocardial infarction and stroke in patients treated with rofecoxib,[13] valdecoxib,[14] and celecoxib,[15] suggesting potential for a mechanism-based cardiovascular hazard for the class, ie, selective COX-2 inhibitors (although not equal for all agents).[16]

Blood Pressure, Renal, and Renovascular Adverse Events

Traditional NSAIDs and COX-2 inhibitors have been associated with renal and renovascular adverse events.[17] NSAIDs have little effect on renal function or blood pressure in normal human subjects. However, in patients with congestive heart failure, hepatic cirrhosis, chronic kidney disease, hypovolemia, and other states of activation of the sympathoadrenal or renin-angiotensin systems, prostaglandin formation and effects in renal blood flow/renal function becomes significant in both model systems and in humans.[18]

Analgesic Nephropathy

Analgesic nephropathy is a condition of slowly progressive renal failure, decreased concentrating capacity of the renal tubule, and sterile pyuria. Risk factors are the chronic use of high doses of combinations of NSAIDs and frequent urinary tract infections. If recognized early, discontinuation of NSAIDs permits recovery of renal function.

Hypersensitivity

Certain individuals display hypersensitivity to aspirin and NSAIDs, as manifested by symptoms that range from vasomotor rhinitis with profuse watery secretions, angioedema, generalized urticaria, and bronchial asthma to laryngeal edema, bronchoconstriction, flushing, hypotension, and shock. Aspirin intolerance is a contraindication to therapy with any other NSAID because cross-sensitivity can provoke a life-threatening reaction reminiscent of anaphylactic shock. Despite the resemblance to anaphylaxis, this reaction does not appear to be immunological in nature.

Although less common in children, this syndrome may occur in 10% to 25% of patients with asthma, nasal polyps, or chronic urticaria, and in 1% of apparently healthy individuals.

Pharmacokinetics and Pharmacodynamics

Most of the NSAIDs are rapidly and completely absorbed from the gastrointestinal tract, with peak concentrations occurring within 1 to 4 hours. Aspirin begins to acetylate platelets within minutes of reaching the presystemic circulation. The presence of food tends to delay absorption without affecting peak concentration. Most NSAIDs are extensively protein-bound (95% to 99%) and undergo hepatic metabolism and renal excretion. In general, NSAIDs are not recommended in the setting of advanced hepatic or renal disease due to their adverse pharmacodynamic effects (**Tables 2 and 3**).

SELECTED NONOPIOID ANALGESICS: CLINICAL PEARLS
Salicylates

Salicylates include acetylated aspirin (acetylsalicylic acid) and the modified salicylate diflunisal, which is a diflurophenyl derivative of salicylic acid. Aspirin was invented in 1897; it is one of the oldest nonopioid oral analgesics. Gastric disturbances and bleeding are common adverse effects with therapeutic doses of aspirin. Because of the possible association with Reye's syndrome, aspirin should not be used for children younger than the age of 12 with viral illness, particularly influenza.

Table 2
Nonopioid analgesics: comparative pharmacology

Drug	Proprietary Names (not all-inclusive)	Average Oral Analgesic Dose, Mg	Dose Interval, h	Maximal Daily Dose, Mg	Analgesic Efficacy Compared to Standards	Plasma Half-Life, h	Comments
Acetaminophen	Numerous	500–1,000	4–6	4000	Comparable to aspirin	2–3	Rectal suppository available for children and adults. Sustained-release preparation available. >2g/d may increase INR in patients receiving Warfarin.
Salicylates	Numerous	500–1000	4–6	4000		0.25	Because of risk of Reye's syndrome, do not use in children under 12 with possible viral illness. Rectal suppository available for children and adults. Sustained-release preparation available.
Acetylated Aspirin							
Modified Diflunisal	Dolobid	1000 initial, 500 subsequent	8–12	1500	500 mg superior to aspirin 650 mg, with slower onset and longer duration; an initial dose of 1000 mg significantly shortens time to onset	8–12	Dose in elderly 500–1000 mg/d
Salicylate salts Choline magnesium	Trilisate	1000–1500	12	2000–3000	Longer duration of action than aspirin 650 mg	9–17	Does not yield salicylate Unlike aspirin and NSAIDs, does not increase bleeding time
Trisalicylate	Tricosal						

NSAIDs	Brand names	Dose (mg)	Duration (h)	Max daily dose (mg)	Analgesic efficacy	Half-life (h)	Comments
Propionic acids							
Ibuprofen	Motrin, Rufen, Nuprin, Advil, Medipren, others	200–400	4–6	2400	Superior at 200 mg to aspirin 650 mg	2–2.5	Most commonly used NSAID in US. Available without prescription.
Naproxen	Naprosyn, Naprolan	500 initial, 250 subsequent	6–8	1500	—	12–15	Better tolerated than indomethacin and aspirin.
Naproxen sodium	Anaprox	550 initial, 275 subsequent	6–8	1650	275 mg comparable to aspirin, 650 mg, with slower onset and longer duration; 550 mg superior to aspirin 650 mg		
Naproxen sodium	Aleve	220 mg	8–12	—	Comparable to aspirin	2–3	—
Fenoprofen	Nalfon	200	4–6	3200	Superior at 25 mg to aspirin 650 mg	1.5	Sustained-release preparation available
Ketoprofen	Orudis	25–50	6–8	300			
Ketoprofen OTC	Actron, Orudis-K+	12.5–25	4–6	—			
Oxaprozin	Daypro	600	12–24	1200		24–69	
Indolacetic acids							
Indomethacin	Indocin, Indocin SR, Indochron E-R				Comparable to aspirin 650 mg	2	Not routinely used because of high incidence of gastrointestinal and Central nervous system side effects; rectal and sustained-release oral forms available for adults

Table 3
Selected nonopioid analgesics: analgesic dosage and comparative efficacy to standards

Drug	Proprietary Names (not all-inclusive)	Average Oral Analgesic Dose, mg	Dose Interval, h	Maximal Daily Dose, mg	Analgesic Efficacy Compared to Standards	Plasma Half-life, h	Comments
Sulindac	Clinoril	150	12	400		7.8 Activemeta = 16	
Etodolac	Lodine	300–400	8–12	1000	More potent than sulindac and naproxen, but less potent than indomethacin		
Pyrrolacetic acids							
Ketorolac	Toradol	30 or 60 mg IM or 30 mg IV initial, 15 or 30 mg IV or IM subsequent	6	150 first d, 120 thereafter	In the range of 6–12 mg of morphine	6	Limit treatment to 5 d; may precipitate renal faiure in dehydrated patients, average dose in elderly 10–15 mg IM/IV Q6 h
Tolmetin	Tolectin	200–600	8	1800		5	
Anthranilic acids							
Mefenamic acid	Ponstel	500 initial, 250 subsequent	6	1500	Comparable to aspirin 650 mg	2	In US use is restricted to interval of 1 wk

Drug	Brand	Dose	Duration (h)	Max	Comments	Half-life	Notes
Phenylacetic acids							
Diclofenac potassium	Cataflam	50 mg	8	150	Superior in efficacy and analgesic duration to aspirin 650 mg		More selective for COX-2 than COX-1
Enolic acids							
Meloxicam	Mobic	7.5–15	24	15		15–20	Ten-fold selective for COX-2
Piroxicam	Feldene	20–40	24	40		50	
Naphthylalkanone							
Nabumetone	Relafen	1000 initial 500–750 subsequent	8–12	2000	Pain relief equal to aspirin, indomethacin, naproxen, and sulindac	24	Fewer gastrointestinal side effects
Cox-2 selective							
Celecoxib	Celebrex	200–400	12–24	400	Anti-inflammatory and analgesic effect similar to naproxen	11	
Rofecoxib	Vioxx	12.5–50	24	25 50 up to 5 d		17	
Valdecoxib	Bextra	10–20	12–24	40		8–11	

Salicylate Salts (Nonacetylated)

Salicylate salts such as choline magnesium trisalicylate and salsalate are effective analgesics and produce fewer GI side effects than aspirin.[19] Unlike aspirin and other nonselective NSAIDs, therapeutic doses do not greatly affect bleeding time or platelet aggregation tests in patients without prior clotting abnormalities.[20]

Acetaminophen

Acetaminophen is a nonsalicylate that may produce similar analgesic and antipyretic potency as aspirin, but has no antiplatelet effects, lacks clinically useful peripheral anti-inflammatory effects, and does not damage the gastric mucosa. Although acetaminophen is well tolerated at recommended doses of up to 4000 mg/d, acute overdoses can cause potentially fatal hepatic necrosis. Patients with chronic alcoholism and liver disease and patients who are fasting can develop severe hepatotoxicity, even at usual therapeutic doses.[21] The Food and Drug Administration (FDA) now requires alcohol warnings for acetaminophen as well as all other nonprescription analgesics.[22] Acetaminophen overdoses are common because acetaminophen is a frequent ingredient in many nonprescription and prescription analgesic formulations. Acetaminophen has a reduced risk of ulcers and ulcer complications when compared with nonselective NSAIDs and is rarely associated with renal toxicity. Acetaminophen is an underrecognized cause of over-anticoagulation with warfarin in the outpatient setting.[23]

Pyrrolacetic Acids

Ketorolac is a pyrrolacetic acid, which is available in injection form. An initial dose of 30 mg followed by 10 to 15 mg intravenously (IV) every 6 hours is equianalgesic to 6 to 12 mg of IV morphine. Ketorolac may precipitate renal failure especially in elderly and hypovolemic patients. It is therefore recommended to limit use of Ketorolac to 5 days only. Also, clinicians should try to use the lowest dose felt to be needed.

Phenylacetic Acid

Diclofenac potassium has been shown to be superior in efficacy and analgesic duration to aspirin and also inhibits selectively more COX-2 then COX-1.

Enolic Acids

Meloxicam has long half-life and roughly 10-fold COX-2 selectivity on average in ex vivo assays.[24] There is significantly less gastric injury compared with piroxicam (20 mg/d) in subjects treated with 7.5 mg/d of meloxicam, but the advantage is lost with 15 mg/d.[25]

Naphthylalkanone

Nabumetone is a prodrug; it is absorbed rapidly and is converted in the liver to one or more active metabolites, principally 6-methoxy-2-naphtylacetic acid, a potent nonselective inhibitor of COX.[26] The incidence of gastrointestinal ulceration appears to be lower than with other NSAIDs [27] (perhaps because of its being a prodrug or the fact that there is essentially no enterohepatic circulation).

Propionic Acids

Ibuprofen and naproxen are the most commonly used NSAIDs in the United States. These are available without a prescription in the United States. The relative risk of myocardial infarction appears unaltered by ibuprofen, but it is reduced by around 10% with naproxen, compared with a reduction of 20% to 25% by aspirin. Ibuprofen and naproxen are better tolerated than aspirin and indomethacin and have been used in patients with a history of gastrointestinal intolerance to other NSAIDs.

Indolacetic Acids

Indomethacin is a more potent inhibitor of the cyclooxygenase than is aspirin, but patient intolerance generally limits its use to short-term dosing. A very high percentage (35% to 50%) of patients receiving usual therapeutic doses of indomethacin experience untoward symptoms. CNS side effects, indeed the most common side effects, include severe frontal headache, dizziness, vertigo, and light-headedness; mental confusion and seizure may also occur, severe depression, psychosis, hallucinations, and suicide have also been reported. Caution must be exercised when starting indomethacin in elderly patients, or patients with history of epilepsy, psychiatric disorders, or Parkinson's disease, because they are greater risk of CNS adverse effects.

COX-2 Selective Inhibitors

Three members of the initial class of COX-2 inhibitors, the coxibs, were approved for use in the United States. Both rofecoxib and valdecoxib have now been withdrawn from the market in view of their adverse event profile. Valdecoxib has been associated with a threefold increase in cardiovascular risk in two studies of patients undergoing cardiovascular bypass graft surgery.[28] Based on interim analysis of data from the Adenomatous Polyp Prevention on Vioxx (APPROVe) study, which showed a significant (twofold) increase in the incidence of serious thromboembolic events in subjects receiving 25 mg of rofecoxib relative to placebo,[13] rofecoxib was withdrawn from the market worldwide.[29] The FDA advisory panel agreed that rofecoxib increased the risk of myocardial infarction and stroke and that the evidence accumulated was more substantial than for valdecoxib and appeared more convincing than for celecoxib. Effects attributed to inhibition of prostaglandin production in the kidney (hypertension and edema) may occur with nonselective COX inhibitors and also with celecoxib. Studies in mice and some epidemiological evidence suggest that the likelihood of hypertension on NSAIDs reflects the degree of inhibition of COX-2 and the selectivity with which it is attained. Thus, the risk of thrombosis, hypertension, and accelerated atherogenesis may be mechanistically integrated. The coxibs should be avoided in patients prone to cardiovascular or cerebrovascular disease. None of the coxibs has established clinical efficacy over NSAIDs. While selective COX-2 inhibitors do not interact to prevent the antiplatelet effect of aspirin, it now is thought that they may lose some of their gastrointestinal advantage over NSAIDs alone when used in conjunction with aspirin.

SUMMARY

NSAIDs are useful analgesics for many pain states, especially those involving inflammation. Their use is frequently overlooked in patients with postoperative and chronic pain. Unless there is a contraindication, the use of an NSAID should be routinely considered to manage acute pain, chronic cancer, and noncancer pain.

REFERENCES

1. Acute Pain Management Guideline Panel. Acute pain management: operative or medical procedures and trauma: clinical practice guidelines. Rockville (MD): Agency for Healthcare Policy and Research, Public Health Service, US Department of Health and Human Services; 1992.
2. Carr D, Goudas L. Acute pain. Lancet 1999;353:2051–8.

3. Zuckerman L, Ferrante F. Nonopioid and opioid analgesics. In: Ashburn M, Rice L, editors. The management of pain. Philadelphia (PA): Churchill-Livingstone; 1998. p. 111–40.

4. McCormack K. Non-steroidal anti-inflammatory drugs and spinal nociceptive processing. Pain 1994;59:9–43.

5. Vane J. Inhibition of prostaglandin synthesis as a mechanism of action for aspirin-like drugs. Nature 1971;234:231–8.

6. Malmberg A, Yaksh T. Hyperalgesia mediated by spinal glutamate or substance P receptor blocked by spinal cyclooxygenase inhibition. Science 1992;257:1276–9.

7. Chandrasekharan N, Dai H, Roos K, et al. COX-3, a cyclooxygenase-1 variant inhibited by acetaminophen and other analgesic/antipyretic drugs: cloning, structure, and expression. Proc Natl Acad Sci U S A 2002;99:13926–31.

8. Deeks JJ, Smith LA, Bradley MD. Efficacy, tolerability, and upper gastrointestinal safety of celecoxib for treatment of osteoarthritis and rheumatoid arthritis: systematic review of randomised controlled trials. BMJ 2002;325:619–26.

9. Rostom A, Dube C, Wells G, et al. Prevention of NSAID-induced gastroduodenal ulcers. Cochrane Database Syst Rev 2002;4:CD002296.

10. McAdam BF, Catella-Lawson F, Mardini IA, et al. Systemic biosynthesis of prostacyclin by cyclooxygenase (cox)-2: the human pharmacology of a selective inhibitor of COX-2. Proc Natl Acad Sci U S A 1999;96:272–7.

11. Catella-Lawson F, McAdam B, Morrison BW, et al. Effects of specific inhibition of cyclooxygenase-2 on sodium balance, hemodynamics, and vasoactive eicosanoids. J Pharmacol Exp Ther 1999;289:735–41.

12. FitzGerald GA. COX-2 and beyond: approaches to prostaglandin inhibition in human disease. Nat Rev Drug Discov 2003;2:879–90.

13. Bresalier RS, Sandler RS, Quan H, et al. Cardiovascular events associated with rofecoxib in a colorectal adenoma chemoprevention trial. N Engl J Med 2005; 352:1092–102.

14. Nussmeier NA, Whelton AA, Brown MT, et al. Complications of COX-2 inhibitors parecoxib and valdecoxib after cardiac surgery. N Engl J Med 2005;352: 1081–91.

15. Solomon SD, McMurray JV, Pfeffer MA, et al. Cardiovascular risk associated with celecoxib in a clinical trial for colorectal adenoma prevention. N Engl J Med 2005; 352:1071–80.

16. Pitt B, Pepine C, Willerson JT. Cyclooxygenase-2 inhibition and cardiovascular events. Circulation 2002;106:167–9.

17. Cheng HF, Harris RC. Cyclooxygenases, the kidney, and hypertension. Hypertension 2004;43:525–30.

18. Patrono C, Dunn MJ. The clinical significance of inhibition of renal prostaglandin synthesis. Kidney Int 1987;32:1–12.

19. Ehrlich G. Primary drug therapy: aspirin vs. the nonsteroidal anti-inflammatory drugs. Postgrad Med 1983;May Spec:9–17.

20. Stuart JJ, Pisko EJ. Choline magnesium trisalicylate does not impair platelet aggregation. Pharmatherapeutica 1981;2(8):547–51.

21. Whitcomb D, Block G. Association of acetaminophen hepatotoxicity with fasting and ethanol use. JAMA 1994;272:1845–50.

22. Food and Drug Administration. Over-the-counter drug products containing analgesic/antipyretic active ingredients for internal use; required alcohol warning; final rule; compliance date. Food and Drug Administration, HHS, Fed Regist 1999;64(51):13066–7.

23. Hylek E, Heiman H, Skates S, et al. Acetaminophen and other risk factors for excessive warfarin anticoagulation. JAMA 1998;279:657–62.
24. Panara MR, Renda G, Sciulli MG, et al. Dose-dependent inhibition of platelet cyclooxygenase-1 and monocyte cyclooxygenase-2 by meloxicam in healthy subjects. J Pharmacol Exp Ther 1999;290:276–80.
25. Patoia L, Santucci L, Furno P, et al. A 4-week, double-blind, parallel-group study to compare the gastrointestinal effects of meloxicam 7.5 mg, meloxicam 15 mg, piroxicam 20 mg and placebo by means of faecal blood loss, endoscopy and symptom evaluation in healthy volunteers. B Brit J Rheumatol 1996;35:61–7.
26. Patrignani P, Panara MR, Greco A, et al. Biochemical and pharmacological characterization of the cyclooxygenase activity of human blood prostaglandin endoperoxide synthases. J Pharmacol Exp Ther 1994;271:1705–12.
27. Scott DL, Palmer RH. Safety and efficacy of nabumetone in osteoarthritis: emphasis on gastrointestinal safety. Aliment Pharmacol Ther 2000;14:443–52.
28. Furberg CD, Psaty BM, FitzGerald GA. Parecoxib, valdecoxib and cardiovascular risk. Circulation 2005;111:249.
29. FitzGerald GA. Coxibs and cardiovascular disease. N Engl J Med 2004;351: 1709–11.

Topical Analgesics

Gary McCleane, MD

KEYWORDS

• Analgesics • Anesthetics • Medication

Among the drugs with well-known peripheral effects are nonsteroidal anti-inflammatory drugs (NSAIDs), local anesthetics, and capsaicin. Less well appreciated is the fact that nitrates, tricyclic antidepressants (TCAs), glutamate receptor antagonists, α-adrenoerecptor antagonists, and cannabinoids may have an analgesic effect when applied topically. The rational for the analgesic effects of these compounds, when applied topically, is discussed in this article.

To patients, it makes sense to apply pain relief directly to where they feel pain. They "know" that oral medication can produce side effects, whereas topical agents are less likely to do so. Knowledgeable physicians, however, understand that pain is influenced by peripheral and central factors. They understand that significant opportunity exists to augment inhibitory or to lessen facilitatory influences on the pain stimulus, and therefore, in general, seem to prefer systemically active agents. Increasing evidence, however, backed up by clinical use, now suggests that topically applied medication can be at least as effective as that administered by the oral route and, in general, has a more favorable side effect profile than orally active agents. In this article, the author looks at medications that have a tradition of topical use and at newer additions to this range of drugs. Although a rich variety of potential pharmacologic targets exists peripherally, to date, only some of these are amenable to currently available therapeutic entities; it is on these that concentration is focused.

Not all medication applied to the skin has a local, peripheral action. Drugs such as fentanyl and buprenorphine, which can be applied to the skin, have predominately central effects. This type of administration is known as "transdermal" to distinguish it from the "topical" analgesics—drugs that are applied to skin and have a predominate peripheral effect.

ANTI-INFLAMMATORY AGENTS
Nonsteroidal Anti-Inflammatory Drugs

Among the most widely used topical agents are the NSAIDs. These agents are known to reduce the production of prostaglandins that sensitize nerve endings at the site of injury. This effect occurs due to the inhibition of the cyclooxygenase (COX) enzyme

This article originally appeared in *Medical Clinics of North America*, Volume 91, Issue 1.
Rampark Pain Centre, 2 Rampark Dromore Road, Lurgan BT66 7JH, Northern Ireland, UK
E-mail address: gary@mccleane.freeserve.co.uk

Perioperative Nursing Clinics 4 (2009) 391–403
doi:10.1016/j.cpen.2009.09.006   **periopnursing.theclinics.com**

that converts arachidonic acid liberated from the phospholipid membrane by phospholipases to prostanoids such as prostaglandin. At least two forms of COX are thought to be important. COX1 is normally expressed in tissues such as stomach and kidneys and plays a physiologic role in maintaining tissue integrity.[1] A second form, COX2, plays a role in pain and inflammation.[1] The analgesic effects of NSAIDs can be dissociated from anti-inflammatory effects, and this may reflect additional spinal and supraspinal actions of NSAIDs to inhibit various aspects of central pain processing.[2] Recent evidence suggests that a third COX, COX3, which is predominately centrally distributed, may also be involved in NSAID or acetaminophen action;[3] however, its role remains uncertain.

When NSAIDs are applied topically, bioavailability and plasma concentrations are 5% to 15% of those achieved by systemic delivery.[4] In human experimental pain models, topically applied NSAIDs produce analgesia in models of cutaneous pain,[5–8] and muscle pain.[9] In terms of clinical use, three major reviews—one examining use in musculoskeletal and soft tissue pain,[10] another looking at data accrued in over 10,000 patients in 86 trials,[11] and the last looking primarily at chronic rheumatic disease[4]—concluded that there was clear and significant evidence that topical NSAIDs have pain-relieving properties.

When NSAIDs are applied topically, relatively high concentrations occur in the dermis, whereas levels in adjacent muscle are as high as when the NSAID is given systemically.[4] Gastrointestinal side effects occur less frequently than when the drug is given orally but are still more likely in patients who have previously demonstrated such responses to oral medication.[10]

Perhaps the greatest danger of topical NSAID use is the risk of polypharmacy. A number of over-the-counter topical and oral NSAIDs are now available, and the risk of overdosing with several different preparations taken at the same time and all containing NSAID is very real.

Nitrates

Conventionally used in the treatment of ischemic heart disease, it now seems that nitrates also have potent analgesic and anti-inflammatory effects. It is known that exogenous nitrates stimulate the release of nitric oxide (NO).[12] This substance is known to be a potent mediator in a wide variety of different cellular systems such as the endothelium and the central and peripheral nervous system. It is released from the endothelium and from neutrophils and macrophages—all known to be intimately involved in the inflammatory process. It appears that NO exerts its effect by stimulating increases in guanylate cyclase, thereby increasing levels of $3',5'$-cyclic GMP.[13] Cholinergic drugs such as acetylcholine produce analgesia in a similar fashion by releasing NO and increasing NO at the nociceptor level.[14]

In addition to this action, NO may activate ATP-sensitive potassium channels and activate peripheral antinociception.[15] Endogenous NO levels may be increased if glutamate levels are increased.[16] Glutamate is known to be an excitatory amino acid, activating N-methyl-D-aspartate (NMDA) receptors, thereby initiating sensitization and protracting the pain process.

Topical nitrate, in the form of glyceryl trinitrate (GTN), has been shown to effectively reduce the pain of osteoarthritis,[17] supraspinatus tendonitis,[18] and infusion-related thrombophlebitis.[19] In addition, it may reduce the pain and inflammation caused by sclerosant treatment of varicose veins[20] and may even be useful in the treatment of vulvar pain.[21] A number of reports suggest that topical nitrates may enhance the analgesic effectiveness of strong opioids.[22–24] but it is likely that this effect is due to systemic absorption of the nitrate and a consequent central action. The predominant side effect associated with topical nitrate use is headache. Currently, patch formulations deliver a relatively large amount of nitrate and, therefore, the incidence of headache is high. Should lower dose patches become available, the utility of this treatment would be increased. GTN is also available in an ointment formulation. Measurement and consistency of dosing are problematic with the ointment formulation, and because there is only a small difference between a potentially analgesic dose and one that causes headache, GTN ointment use is less practical than the use of the patch varieties.

Topical nitrates can therefore be considered when pain is localized and particularly in patients in whom NSAIDs are contraindicated. Nitrates are devoid of the renal, gastrointestinal, and hematologic side effects of NSAIDs.

LOCAL ANESTHETICS
Gels/creams

Several topical local anesthetic preparations are available in gel, cream, and patch form. Amethocaine is available as a gel and lidocaine/prilocaine is presented as a cream. The cream contains a eutectic mixture of lidocaine and prilocaine and its use has become established in the anesthetizing of skin before cannula insertion. It also has demonstrable benefit in reducing the pain of other procedures including lumbar puncture, intramuscular injections, and circumcision.[25] Although lidocaine/prilocaine cream is not US Food and Drug Administration (FDA) approved for any neuropathic pain condition, several studies have been undertaken in patients who have postherpetic neuralgia (PHN). Two of these studies were uncontrolled and showed a pain-reducing effect,[26,27] whereas a randomized controlled study of the same condition failed to show any benefit.[28] Caution should be used with long-term use of this preparation because prilocaine use has been associated with the onset of methemoglobinemia.

Patches

Lidocaine is available in a topically applied patch at a 5% strength. In the United States, this preparation is approved by the FDA for the treatment of PHN. Its efficacy in this pain condition is supported by several trials that also confirm that it is well tolerated,[29,30] Not only can pain levels in patients who have PHN be reduced but measures of quality of life also show improvement.[31] In one study of patients who had PHN, 66% of subjects reported reduced pain intensity when up to three lidocaine 5% patches were used for 12 hours each day.[31]

Although lidocaine 5% is indicated for use in PHN, it may also be efficacious in other pain conditions. When used in the treatment of focal neuropathic pain conditions such as mononeuropathies and intercostal and ilioinguinal neuralgia, one controlled study confirmed a pain-reducing effect.[32] In an open-label study of 16 patients who had "refractory" neuropathic pain (including patients who had post-thoracotomy pain, complex regional pain syndrome, postamputation pain, neuroma pain, painful diabetic neuropathy, meralgia parasthetica, and postmastectomy pain), 81% of subjects experienced notable pain relief.[33] In this report, *refractory* was defined as those who had failed to gain pain relief or who experienced unacceptable side effects with opiates, anticonvulsants, antidepressants, or antiarrhythmic agents.

CAPSAICIN

Capsaicin use has a long history in medical practice. Extract of chili pepper was reported in the midnineteenth century to reduce chilblain pain and toothache.[34] It has now been shown to reduce the pain associated with painful diabetic neuropathy.[35–38] PHN,[39–41] chronic distal painful polyneuropathy,[42] oral neuropathic pain,[43] surgical neuropathic pain,[44] and the pain associated with Guillain-Barré syndrome.[45] In the treatment of non-neuropathic pain, capsaicin has a role, with evidence of a pain-relieving effect in osteoarthritis,[46–51] and neck pain.[52]

It appears that capsaicin achieves its pain-relieving effect by reversibly depleting sensory nerve endings of substance P[53,54] and by reducing the density of epidermal nerve fibers, also in a reversible fashion.[55]

When used clinically, the major impediment to better compliance is the intense burning sensation associated with capsaicin's use. This sensation generally reduces with repeated administration, although when capsaicin cream is applied outside the normal area of application, discomfort is again apparent. It has been shown that coadministration of GTN can reduce the discomfort associated with application[50,56,57] and enhance the analgesic effect of the capsaicin.[50] Alternatively, preapplication of lidocaine 5% cream can also reduce application-associated discomfort.[58]

Some patients experience bouts of sneezing when capsaicin is used, which is normally caused by overapplication and drying of the cream on the skin and then nasal inhalation of the capsaicin dust from the application site. Care must always be used so that capsaicin is not applied to moist areas because this is associated with increased burning sensation.

TRICYCLIC ANTIDEPRESSANTS

TCAs, when taken orally, have a long pedigree in pain management. Their use is established in a broad range of pain conditions. Their pain-relieving effect is independent of their antidepressant effect. It is unfortunate that their use is also associated with a significant risk of side effects (eg, dry mouth, sedation, urinary retention, and weight gain), which reduces compliance. In contrast, when TCAs are applied topically, side effects are relatively rare, yet a very real chance of pain relief exists. Any relief obtained by topical TCA use can be rationalized by their possible peripheral actions.

Adenosine Receptors

At peripheral nerve terminals in rodents, adenosine A_1 receptor activation produces antinociception by decreasing cyclic AMP levels in the sensory nerve terminals, whereas adenosine A_2 receptor activation produces pronociception by increasing cyclic AMP levels in the sensory nerve terminals. Adenosine A_3 receptor activation produces pain behaviors due to the release of histamine and serotonin from mast cells and subsequent actions in the sensory nerve terminal.[59] Caffeine acts as a nonspecific adenosine receptor antagonist. When systemic caffeine is administered with systemic amitriptyline, the normal effect on thermal hyperalgesia is blocked. When amitriptyline is administered into a rodent paw that has neuropathic pain, an antihyperalgesic effect is recorded (but not when it is given into the contralateral paw). This antihyperalgesic effect is blocked by caffeine,[60] suggesting that at least part of the effect of peripherally applied amitriptyline is mediated through peripheral adenosine receptors.

Sodium Channels

Sudoh and colleagues[61] injected various TCAs by a single injection into rat sciatic notches. These investigators measured the duration of complete sciatic nerve blockade and compared these values with that of bupivacaine. They found that amitriptyline, doxepin, and imipramine produced a longer complete sciatic nerve block than bupivacaine, whereas trimipramine and desipramine produced a shorter block. Nortriptyline and maprotiline failed to produce any block. When the effect of topical application of amitriptyline is compared with that of lidocaine, amitriptyline is seen to produce longer cutaneous analgesia.[62]

These studies suggest, therefore, that from a mode-of-action perspective, TCAs could have an analgesic effect when applied peripherally.

Animal Evidence of an Antinociceptive Effect of Peripherally Applied Tricyclic Antidepressants

Neuropathic pain
When amitriptyline is applied to rodent paws made neuropathic by a chronic nerve constriction injury, an antinociceptive effect is observed. When the amitriptyline is applied to the contralateral paw, no antinociceptive effect is observed in the paw on the injured side[63,64] When desipramine and the selective serotonin reuptake inhibitor fluoxetine are considered, desipramine has a similar antinociceptive effect when applied topically, whereas fluoxetine does not.[65]

Formalin test
It seems that when amitriptyline[66-68] and desipramine[65] are coadministered peripherally with formalin, the first- and second-phase responses are reduced.

When amitriptyline is administered peripherally along with formalin, Fos immunoreactivity in the dorsal region of the spinal cord is significantly lower than in animals in which formalin is administered alone.[68]

Visceral pain
Using a noxious colorectal distension model in the rat, Su and Gebhart[69] showed that the antidepressants imipramine, desipramine, and clomipramine reduce the response to noxious colorectal distension by 20%, 22%, and 46%, respectively, compared with control-treated animals.

Thermal injury
Thermal hyperalgesia is produced by exposing a rodent hindpaw to 52°C for 45 seconds. Locally applied amitriptyline at the time of thermal injury may produce antihyperalgesic and analgesic effects, depending on the concentration used. When the amitriptyline is applied after the injury, the analgesic effect, but not the antihyperalgesic effect, is retained.[70]

Human pain
Human evidence of an analgesic effect with the topical application of TCAs is limited. A small randomized, placebo-controlled trial of 40 subjects who had neuropathic pain of mixed etiology produced a reduction of 1.18 on a 0-to-10 linear visual analog score relative to placebo use with the application of a doxepin 5% cream. Minor side effects were seen in only 3 subjects.[71] A larger randomized controlled trial involving 200 subjects, again with neuropathic pain of mixed etiology, suggested that doxepin 5% cream reduced the linear visual analog score by about 1 relative to placebo and that time to effect was about 2 weeks. Again, side effects were minor and infrequent.[72] A pilot study examining the effect of topical amitriptyline application failed to produce any pain relief, but the maximum therapy duration was 7 days;[73] the study may have been terminated before the time to maximal effect had been reached.

Case reports have been made of a useful reduction in pain when doxepin 5% cream was applied topically in subjects who had complex regional pain syndrome type I[74] and when doxepin was used as an oral rinse in patients who had oral pain as a result of cancer or cancer therapy.[75]

Although the human evidence of an analgesic effect with topical doxepin is interesting, more study is needed to verify its effects and the effects of other TCAs when used by this route of administration. Evidence suggests that the effect of topically applied doxepin is a local effect and that the consequences of systemic administration and, hence, systemic side effects can be substantially reduced. Doxepin in a 5% cream formulation is currently available and is indicated in the treatment of itch associated with eczema.

GLUTAMATE RECEPTOR ANTAGONIST

It has recently become apparent that glutamate receptors are expressed on peripheral nerve terminals and that these may contribute to peripheral nociceptive signaling. Ionotropic and metabotropic glutamate receptors are present on membranes of unmyelinated peripheral axons and axon terminals in the skin[76,77] and peripheral inflammation increases the proportions of unmyelinated and myelinated nerves expressing ionotropic glutamate receptors.[78] Local injections of NMDA and non-NMDA glutamate receptor agonists to the rat hindpaw,[79,80] or knee joint[81] enhance pain behaviors generating hyperalgesia and allodynia. Injections of metabotropic glutamate receptor agonists produce similar actions[76,82] Local application of glutamate receptor antagonists inhibits pain behavior following formalin application.[81]

In humans, ketamine, a noncompetitive NMDA receptor antagonist, enhances the local anesthetic and analgesic effects of bupivicaine in acute postoperative pain by a peripheral mechanism.[83] When a thermal injury was inflicted in volunteers, one study suggested that subcutaneous injection of ketamine produces long-lasting reduction in hyperalgesia,[84] whereas another study failed to confirm this result.[85] That said, not only may any analgesic effect produced by peripheral ketamine application be due to its glutamate receptor activity but ketamine may also block voltage-sensitive calcium channels, alter cholinergic and monoaminergic actions, and interfere with opioid receptors.[86–88]

Isolated case reports suggest that topical ketamine can reduce sympathetically maintained pain[89] and pain of malignant origin,[90] again suggesting that perhaps glutamate receptor antagonists may have some analgesic effect when applied topically.

α-ADRENORECEPTOR ANTAGONISTS

Clonidine, an α_2-adrenoreceptor agonist can be obtained in cream and patch formulations. It can have peripheral and central action when applied topically. Clonidine patches have been reported to reduce the hyperalgesia associated with sympathetically maintained pain but not the hyperalgesia in patients who have sympathetically independent pain.[91] Clonidine cream may also have some pain-relieving effect in orofacial neuralgia-like pain.[92] The effect of clonidine in sympathetically maintained pain may be related to its effect of reducing presynaptic norepinephrine release from sympathetic nerves. In patients who have sympathetically maintained pain, localized norepinephrine injection worsens the mechanical and thermal hyperalgesia in some.[93,94] and in those who have peripheral nerve injury[95] and PHN.[96]

When clonidine is injected into the knee joint after arthroscopy, pain relief is observed;[97,98] when injected along with bupivicain[99,100] and morphine,[101] the analgesic effect of these drugs is enhanced.

CANNABINOIDS

Cannabinoids (CBs) can act at peripheral sites to produce analgesia by virtue of their effect on CB_1 and CB_2 receptors. In animal models, peripheral administration of agents selective for CB_1 receptors produces local analgesia in the formalin test,[102] the carrageenan hyperalgesia model,[103] and the nerve injury model.[104] This effect may be obtained because of the effects of these agents on the sensory nerve terminal to inhibit release of calcitonin gene–related peptide[103] or by inhibiting effects of nerve growth factor.[105] CB_2 receptor mechanisms may play a prominent role in inflammatory pain.[105]

OPIOIDS

The analgesic effects of systemic opioids are well established and beyond question. Recently, transdermal formulations of fentanyl and buprenorphine have been introduced. Although they are applied to skin, it is likely that their predominant effect is central.

It is now apparent that opioid receptors are not exclusively located in the central nervous system. It appears that opioid receptors are synthesized in dorsal root ganglia and transported into peripheral terminals of primary afferent neurons[106,107] Both mu and delta opioid receptors can be identified in fine cutaneous nerves in opioid-naïve animals.[108] When a ligature is placed on the rat sciatic nerve, β-endorphin binding sites accumulate proximally and distally to the ligature site.[109] When inflammation is induced, the number of β-endorphin binding sites on both sides of the ligature massively increases.[109]

From the human clinical perspective, a number of reports suggest that the knowledge of a peripheral representation of opioid receptors may have practical application. Topical morphine, provided as an oral rinse, has been shown to reduce mucositis-related pain in patients undergoing chemotherapy for head and neck carcinomas.[110,111] whereas other case reports suggest that topical opioids may reduce pain from skin ulcer[112,113] In patients undergoing dental extractions, mixed results have been obtained, with some reporting enhanced relief when morphine is applied locally after dental extraction.[114,115] and others reporting no such effect.[116] It has also been suggested that intravesical, strong opioids can reduce painful bladder spasms[117,118]

Despite these suggestions from the literature, two systematic reviews failed to find any evidence of a pain-relieving effect when morphine was used by peripheral application.[119,120]

SUMMARY

Our knowledge and understanding of the pathophysiology and treatment of pain is increasing; however, we should not lose sight of the simple opportunities that exist for intercepting pain at peripheral targets. Although systemic medication often has peripheral and central modes of action, the appeal for provision of medication close to where these peripheral targets exist should be high. If these sites can be attacked with relatively high concentrations of active drug while keeping systemic levels of that drug below the level at which systemic side effects become apparent, then this should lead to desirable outcomes. Even though the number of true topical agents with an indication for this use is small, a number of other topical agents are available that evidence suggests have the possibility of being effective. Given the increased understanding of pain, the likelihood of further topical agents becoming available is high.

REFERENCES

1. Vane JR, Bakhle YS, Botting J. Cyclo-oxygenase 1 and 2. Annu Rev Pharmacol Toxicol 1998;38:97–120.

2. Yaksh TL, Dirig DM, Malmberg AB. Mechanisms of action of nonsteroidal anti-inflammatory drugs. Cancer Investig 1998;16:509–27.
3. Chandrasekharan NV, Dai H, Roos KL, et al. Cox-3, a cyclo-oxygenase-1 variant inhibited by acetaminophen and other analgesic/antipyretic drugs. Cloning, structure and expression. Proc Natl Acad Sci U S A 2002;99:13926–31.
4. Heyneman CA, Lawless-Liday C, Wall GC. Oral versus topical NSAIDs in rheumatic diseases. A comparison. Drugs 2000;60:555–74.
5. Kress M, Reeh PW. Chemical excitation and sensitization in nociceptors. In: Cavero F, Belmonte C, editors. Neurobiology and nociceptors. Oxford (UK): Oxford University Press; 1996. p. 258–97.
6. Steen KH, Reeh PW, Kreysel HW. Topical acetylsalicylic, salicylic acid and indomethacin suppresses pain from experimental tissue acidosis in human skin. Pain 1995;62:339–47.
7. Steen KH, Reeh PW, Kreysel HW. Dose-dependent competitive block by topical acetylsalicylic acid and salicylic acid of low pH-induced cutaneous pain. Pain 2001;64:71–82.
8. Schmelz M, Kress M. Topical acetylsalicylate attenuates capsaicin induced pain, flare and allodynia but not thermal hyperalgesia. Neurosci Lett 1996;214:72–4.
9. Steen KH, Wegner H, Meller ST. Analgesic profile of peroral and topical ketoprofen upon low pH-induced muscle pain. Pain 2001;93:23–33.
10. Vaile JH, Davis P. Topical NSAIDs for musculoskeletal conditions. A review of the literature. Drugs 1998;56:783–99.
11. Moore RA, Tramer MR, Carrol D, et al. Quantitative systematic review of topically applied non-steroidal anti-inflammatory drugs. BMJ 1998;316:333–8.
12. Feelisch M, Noack EA. Correlation between nitric oxide formation during degradation of organic nitrates and activation of guanylate cyclase. Eur J Pharmacol 1987;139:19–30.
13. Knowles RG, Palacios M, Palmer RM, et al. Formation of nitric oxide from L-arginine in the central nervous system: a transduction mechanism for stimulation of soluble guanylate cyclase. Proc Natl Acad Sci U S A 1989;86:5159–62.
14. Duarte ID, Lorenzetti BB, Ferreira SH. Acetylcholine induces peripheral analgesia by the release of nitric oxide. In: Moncada S, Higgs A, editors. Nitric oxide from L-arginine. A bioregulatory system. Amsterdam: Elsevier; 1990. p. 165–70.
15. Soares A, Leite R, Patsuo M, et al. Activation of ATP sensitive K channels: mechanisms of peripheral antinociceptive action of the nitric oxide donor, sodium nitroprusside. Eur J Pharmacol 2000;14:67–71.
16. Okuda K, Sakurada C, Takahashi M, et al. Characterization of nociceptive responses and spinal release of nitric oxide metabolites and glutamate evoked by different concentrations of formalin in rats. Pain 2001;92:107–15.
17. McCleane GJ. The addition of piroxicam to topically applied glyceryl trinitrate enhances its analgesic effect in musculoskeletal pain: a randomised, double-blind, placebo-controlled study. Pain Clin 2000;12:113–6.
18. Berrazueta JR, Losada A, Poveda J, et al. Successful treatment of shoulder pain syndrome due to supraspinatus tendonitis with transdermal nitroglycerin. A double blind study. Pain 1996;66:63–7.
19. Berrazeuta JR, Poveda JJ, Ochoteco JA, et al. The anti-inflammatory and analgesic action of transdermal glyceryl trinitrate in the treatment of infusion related thrombophlebitis. Postgrad Med J 1993;69:37–40.
20. Berrazueta JR, Fleitas M, Salas E, et al. Local transdermal glyceryl trinitrate has an anti-inflammatory action on thrombophlebitis induced by sclerosis of leg varicose veins. Angiology 1994;45:347–51.

21. Walsh KE, Berman JR, Berman LA, et al. Safety and efficacy of topical nitroglycerin for treatment of vulvar pain in women with vulvodynia: a pilot study. J Gend Specif Med 2002;5:21–7.
22. Lauretti GR, de Oliveira R, Reis MP, et al. Transdermal nitroglycerine enhances spinal sufentanil postoperative analgesia following orthopaedic surgery. Anesthesiology 1999;90:734–9.
23. Lauretti GR, Lima IC, Reis MP. Oral ketamine and transdermal nitroglycerin as analgesic adjuvants to oral morphine therapy for cancer pain management. Anesthesiology 1999;90:1528–33.
24. Lauretti GR, Perez MV, Reis MP, et al. Double-blind evaluation of transdermal nitroglycerine as an adjuvant to oral morphine for cancer pain management. J Clin Anesth 2002;14:83–6.
25. Galer BS. Topical medications. In: Loeser JD, editor. Bonica's management of pain. Philadelphia: Lippincott-Williams & Wilkins; 2001. p. 1736–41.
26. Attal N, Brasseur L, Chauvin M. Effects of single and repeated applications of a eutectic mixture of local anesthetics (EMLA®) cream on spontaneous and evoked pain in post-herpetic neuralgia. Pain 1999;81:203–9.
27. Litman SJ, Vitkun SA, Poppers PJ. Use of EMLA® cream in the treatment of post-herpetic neuralgia. J Clin Anesth 1996;8:54–7.
28. Lycka BA, Watson CP, Nevin K, et al. EMLA® cream for the treatment of pain caused by post-herpetic neuralgia: a double-blind, placebo controlled study. Proceedings of the Annual Meeting of the American Pain Society. Glenview (IL): American Pain Society; 1996. A111 (abstract).
29. Rowbotham MC, Davies PS, Verkempinck C, et al. Lidocaine patch: double-blind controlled study of a new treatment method for post-herpetic neuralgia. Pain 1996;65:39–44.
30. Galer BS, Rowbotham MC, Perander J, et al. Topical lidocaine patch relieves post-herpetic neuralgia more effectively than vehicle patch: results of an enriched enrolment study. Pain 1999;80:533–8.
31. Katz NP, Davis MW, Dworkin RH. Topical lidocaine patch produces a significant improvement in mean pain scores and pain relief in treated PHN patients: results of a multicenter open-label trial. J Pain 2001;2:9–18.
32. Meier T, Wasner G, Faust M, et al. Efficacy of lidocaine 5% patch in treatment of focal peripheral neuropathic pain syndromes: a randomized, double-blind, placebo-controlled study. Pain 2003;106:151–8.
33. Devers A, Galer BS. Topical lidocaine patch relieves a variety of neuropathic pain conditions: an open-label study. Clin J Pain 2000;16:205–8.
34. Capsaicin Study Group. Treatment of painful diabetic neuropathy with topical capsaicin. Arch Intern Med 1991;151:2225–9.
35. Tandan R, Lewis GA, Krusinski PB, et al. Topical capsaicin in painful diabetic neuropathy. Diabetes Care 1992;15:8–13.
36. Capsaicin Study Group. Effect of treatment with capsaicin on daily activities of patients with painful diabetic neuropathy. Diabetes Care 1992;15: 159–65.
37. Chad DA, Aronin N, Lundstorm R, et al. Does capsaicin relieve the pain of diabetic neuropathy? Pain 1990;42:387–8.
38. Bernstein JE, Korman NJ, Bickers DR, et al. Topical capsaicin treatment of chronic postherpetic neuralgia. J Am Acad Dermatol 1989;21:265–70.
39. Watson CP, Tyler KL, Bickers DR, et al. A randomized vehicle controlled trial of topical capsaicin in the treatment of postherpetic neuralgia. Clin Ther 1993;15: 510–26.

40. Watson CP, Evans R, Watt VR. Post herpetic neuralgia and topical capsaicin. Pain 1988;33:333–40.
41. Low PA, Opfer-Gehrking TL, Dyck PJ, et al. Double blind, placebo controlled study of the application of capsaicin cream in chronic distal painful polyneuropathy. Pain 1995;45:163–8.
42. Epstein JB, Marcoe JH. Topical application of capsaicin for treatment of oral neuropathic pain and trigeminal neuralgia. Oral Surg Oral Med Oral Pathol 1994;77:135–40.
43. Ellison N, Loprinzi CL, Kugler J, et al. Phase III placebo controlled trial of capsaicin cream in the management of surgical neuropathic pain in cancer patients. J Clin Oncol 1997;15:2974–80.
44. Morgenlander JC, Hurwitz BJ, Massey EW. Capsaicin for the treatment of pain in Guillain-Barré syndrome. Ann Neurol 1990;12:199.
45. Turnbull A. Tincture of capsicum as a remedy for chilblains and toothache. Dublin (Ireland): Dublin Medical Press; 1850. p. 95–6.
46. Altman RD, Aven A, Holmburg CE, et al. Capsaicin cream 0.025% as monotherapy for osteoarthritis: a double blind study. Sem Arth Rheum 1994;23S:25–33.
47. Deal CL. The use of topical capsaicin in managing arthritis pain: a clinician's perspective. Sem Arth Rheum 1994;23S:48–52.
48. Deal CL, Schnitzer TJ, Lipstein E, et al. Treatment of arthritis with topical capsaicin: a double blind trial. Clin Ther 1991;13:383–95.
49. McCarthy GM, McCarty DJ. Effect of topical capsaicin in the therapy of painful osteoarthritis of the hands. J Rheumatol 1992;19:604–7.
50. McCleane GJ. The analgesic efficacy of topical capsaicin in enhanced by glyceryl trinitrate in painful osteoarthritis: a randomized, double-blind, placebo controlled study. Eur J Pain 2000;4:355–60.
51. Schnitzer T, Morton C, Coker S. Topical capsaicin therapy for osteoarthritis pain: achieving a maintenance regimen. Sem Arth Rheum 1994;23S:34–40.
52. Mathias BJ, Dillingham TR, Zeigler DN, et al. Topical capsaicin for chronic neck pain. Am J Phys Med Rehabil 1995;74:39–44.
53. Fitzgerald M. Capsaicin and sensory neurones. Pain 1983;15:109–30.
54. Rains C, Bryson HM. Topical capsaicin. A review of its pharmacological properties and therapeutic potential in post herpetic neuralgia, diabetic neuropathy and osteoarthritis. Drugs Aging 1995;7:317–28.
55. Nolano M, Simone DA, Wendelschafer-Crabb G, et al. Topical capsaicin in humans: parallel loss of epidermal nerve fibers and pain sensation. Pain 1999;81:135–41.
56. Walker RA, McCleane GJ. The addition of glyceryl trinitrate to capsaicin cream reduces the thermal allodynia associated with the use of capsaicin in humans. Neurosci Lett 2002;323:78–80.
57. McCleane GJ, McLaughlin M. The addition of GTN to capsaicin cream reduces the discomfort associated with application of capsaicin alone. A volunteer study. Pain 1998;78:149–51.
58. Yosipovitch G, Mailback HI, Rowbotham MC. Effect of EMLA pre-treatment on capsaicin-induced burning and hyperalgesia. Acta Derm Venereol 1999;79:118–21.
59. Sawynok J. Adenosine receptor activation and nociception. Eur J Pharmacol 1998;317:1–11.
60. Esser MJ, Sawynok MJ. Caffeine blockade of the thermal antihyperalgesic effect of acute amitriptyline in a rat model of neuropathic pain. Eur J Pharmacol 2000;399:131–9.

61. Sudoh Y, Cahoon EE, Gerner P, et al. Tricyclic antidepressant as long acting local anesthetics. Pain 2003;103:49–55.
62. Haderer A, Gerner P, Kao G, et al. Cutaneous analgesia after transdermal application of amitriptyline versus lidocaine in rats. Anesth Analg 2003;96:1707–10.
63. Esser MJ, Sawynok J. Acute amitriptyline in a rat model of neuropathic pain: differential symptom and route effects. Pain 1999;80:643–53.
64. Esser MJ, Chase T, Allen GV, et al. Chronic administration of amitriptyline and caffeine in a rat model of neuropathic pain: multiple interactions. Eur J Pharmacol 2001;430:211–8.
65. Sawynok J, Esser MJ, Reid AR. Peripheral antinociceptive actions of desipramine and fluoxetine in an inflammatory and neuropathic pain test in the rat. Pain 1999;82:149–58.
66. Sawynok J, Reid AR, Esser MJ. Peripheral antinociceptive action of amitriptyline in the rat formalin test: involvement of adenosine. Pain 1999;80:45–55.
67. Sawynok J, Reid A. Peripheral interactions between dextromethorphan, ketamine and amitriptyline on formalin-evoked behaviours and paw edema in rats. Pain 2003;102:179–86.
68. Heughan CE, Allen GV, Chase TD, et al. Peripheral amitriptyline suppresses formalin-induced Fos expression in the rat spinal cord. Anesth Analg 2002;94:427–31.
69. Su X, Gebhart GF. Effects of tricyclic antidepressants on mechanosensitive pelvic nerve afferent fibers innervating the rat colon. Pain 1998;76:105–14.
70. Oatway M, Reid A, Sawynok J. Peripheral antihyperalgesic and analgesic actions of ketamine and amitriptyline in a model of mild thermal injury in the rat. Anesth Analg 2003;97:168–73.
71. McCleane GJ. Topical doxepin hydrochloride reduces neuropathic pain: a randomized, double-blind, placebo controlled study. Pain Clin 1999;12:47–50.
72. McCleane GJ. Topical application of doxepin hydrochloride, capsaicin and a combination of both produces analgesia in chronic human neuropathic pain: a randomized, double-blind, placebo-controlled study. Br J Clin Pharmacol 2000;49:574–9.
73. Lynch ME, Clarke AJ, Sawynok J. A pilot study examining topical amitriptyline, ketamine, and a combination of both in the treatment of neuropathic pain. Clin J Pain 2003;19:323–8.
74. McCleane GJ. Topical application of doxepin hydrochloride can reduce the symptoms of complex regional pain syndrome: a case report. Injury 2002;33:88–9.
75. Epstein JB, Truelove EL, Oien H, et al. Oral topical doxepin rinse: analgesic effect in patients with oral mucosal pain due to cancer or cancer therapy. Oral Oncol 2001;37:632–7.
76. Zhou S, Komak S, Du J, et al. Metabotropic glutamate 1α receptors on peripheral primary afferent fibers: their role in nociception. Brain Res 2001;913:18–26.
77. Carlton SM, Hargett GL, Coggeshall RE. Localization and activation of glutamate receptors in unmyelinated axons of rat glabrous skin. Neurosci Lett 1995;197:25–8.
78. Carlton SM, Coggeshall RE. Inflammation-induced changes in peripheral glutamate receptor populations. Brain Res 1999;820:63–70.
79. Zhou S, Bonasera L, Carlton SM. Peripheral administration of NMDA, AMPA or KA results in pain behaviour in rats. Neuroreport 1996;7:895–900.
80. Jackson DL, Graff CB, Richardson JD. Glutamate participates in the peripheral modulation of thermal hyperalgesia in rats. Eur J Pharmacol 1995;284:321–5.

81. Lawland NB, Willis WD, Westlund KN. Excitatory amino acid receptor involvement in peripheral nociceptive transmission in rats. Eur J Pharmacol 1997; 324:169–77.

82. Walker K, Reeve A, Bowes M, et al. mGlu5 receptors and nociceptive function II. mGlu5 receptors functionally expressed on peripheral sensory neurones mediate inflammatory hyperalgesia. Neuropharmacology 2001; 40:10–9.

83. Tverskoy M, Oren M, Vaskovich M, et al. Ketamine enhances local anesthetic and analgesic effects of bupivicaine by a peripheral mechanism: a study in postoperative patients. Neurosci Lett 1996;215:5–8.

84. Warncke T, JØrum E, Stubhaug A. Local treatment with the N-methyl-D-aspartate receptor antagonist ketamine, inhibits development of secondary hyperalgesia in man by a peripheral action. Neurosci Lett 1997;227:1–4.

85. Pedersen JL, Galle TS, Kehlet H. Peripheral analgesic effects of ketamine in acute inflammatory pain. Anesthesiology 1998;89:58–66.

86. Hirota K, Lambert DG. Ketamine: its mechanism(s) of action and unusual clinical uses. Br J Anaesth 1996;77:441–4.

87. Meller ST. Ketamine: relief from chronic pain through actions at the NMDA receptor? Pain 1996;68:435–6.

88. Sawynok J, Reid AR. Modulation of formalin-induced behaviours and edema by local and systemic administration of dextromethorphan, memantine and ketamine. Eur J Pharmacol 2002;450:115–21.

89. Crowley KL, Flores JA, Hughes CN, et al. Clinical application of ketamine ointment in the treatment of sympathetically maintained pain. Int J Pharmaceutical Compounding 1998;2:122–7.

90. Wood RM. Ketamine for pain in hospice patients. Int J Pharmaceutical Compounding 2000;4:253–4.

91. Davis CL, Treede RD, Raja SN, et al. Topical application of clonidine relieves hyperalgesia in patients with sympathetically maintained pain. Pain 1991;47:309–17.

92. Epstein JB, Grushka M, Le N. Topical clonidine for orofacial pain: a pilot study. J Orofac Pain 1997;11:346–52.

93. Torebjörk E, Wahren L, Wallin G, et al. Noradrenaline-evoked pain in neuralgia. Pain 1995;63:11–20.

94. Ali Z, Raja SN, Wesselmann U, et al. Intradermal injection of norepinephrine evokes pain in patients with sympathetically maintained pain. Pain 2000;88:161–8.

95. Chabal C, Jacobson L, Mariano A, et al. The use of oral mexiletine for the treatment of pain after peripheral nerve injury. Anesthesiology 1992;76:513–7.

96. Choi B, Rowbotham MC. Effect of adrenergic receptor activation on postherpetic neuralgia pain and sensory disturbances. Pain 1997;69:55–63.

97. Gentili M, Houssel P, Osman H, et al. Intra-articular morphine and clonidine produce comparable analgesia but the combination is not more effective. Br J Anaesth 1997;79:660–1.

98. Gentili M, Juhel A, Bonnet F. Peripheral analgesic effect of intra-articular clonidine. Pain 1996;64:593–6.

99. Reuben SS, Connelly NR. Postoperative analgesia for outpatient arthroscopic knee surgery with intraarticular clonidine. Anesth Analg 1999;88:729–33.

100. Joshi M, Reuben SS, Kilaru PR, et al. Postoperative analgesia for outpatient arthroscopic knee surgery with intraarticular clonidine and/or morphine. Anesth Analg 2000;90:1102–6.

101. Buerkle H, Huge V, Wolfgart M, et al. Intra-articular clonidine analgesia after knee arthroscopy. Eur J Anaesthesiol 2000;17:295–9.
102. Calignano A, La Ranna G, Giuffrida A, et al. Control of pain initiation by endogenous cannabinoids. Nature 1998;394:277–81.
103. Richardson JD, Kilo S, Hargreaves KM. Cannabinoids reduce hyperalgesia and inflammation via interaction with peripheral CB1 receptors. Pain 1998;75:111–9.
104. Fox A, Kesingland A, Gentry C, et al. The role of central and peripheral cannabinoid$_1$ receptors in the antihyperalgesic activity of cannabinoids in a model of neuropathic pain. Pain 2001;92:91–100.
105. Rice AS, Farquhar-Smith WP, Nagy I. Endocannabinoids and pain: spinal and peripheral analgesia in inflammation and neuropathy. Prostaglandins Leukot Essent Fatty Acids 2002;66:243–56.
106. Zhou L, Zhang Q, Stein C, et al. Contribution of opioid receptors on primary afferent versus sympathetic neurons to peripheral opioid analgesia. J Pharmacol Exp Ther 1998;286:1000–6.
107. Stein C, Schafer H, Hassan AH. Peripheral opioid receptors. Ann Med 1995;27:219–21.
108. Coggeshall RE, Zhou S, Carlton SM. Opioid receptors on peripheral sensory axons. Brain Res 1997;764:126–32.
109. Hassan AH, Ableitner A, Stein C, et al. Inflammation of the rat paw enhances axonal transport of opioid receptors in the sciatic nerve and increases their density in the inflamed tissue. Neuroscience 1993;55:185–95.
110. Cerchietti LC, Navigante AH, Bonomi MR, et al. Effect of topical morphine for mucositis-associated pain following concomitant chemoradiotherapy for head and neck carcinoma. Cancer 2002;95:2230–6.
111. Cerchietti LC, Navigante AH, Körte MW, et al. Potential utility of the peripheral analgesic properties of morphine in stomatitis-related pain: a pilot study. Pain 2003;105:265–73.
112. Krajnik M, Zylicz Z, Finlay I, et al. Potential uses of topical opioids in palliative care—report of 6 cases. Pain 1999;80:121–5.
113. Twillman RK, Long TD, Cathers TA, et al. Treatment of painful skin ulcers with topical opioids. J Pain Symptom Manage 1999;17:288–92.
114. Likar R, Sittl R, Gragger K, et al. Peripheral morphine analgesia in dental surgery. Pain 1998;76:145–50.
115. Likar R, Koppert W, Blatnig H, et al. Efficacy of peripheral morphine analgesia in inflamed, non-inflamed perineural tissue of dental surgery patients. J Pain Symptom Manage 2001;21:330–7.
116. Moore RJ, Seymour RA, Gilro J, et al. The efficacy of locally applied morphine in post-operative pain after bilateral third molar surgery. Br J Clin Pharmacol 1994;37:227–30.
117. Duckett JW, Cangiano T, Cubina M, et al. Intravesical morphine analgesia after bladder surgery. J Urol 1997;157:1407–9.
118. McCoubrie R, Jeffrey D. Intravesical diamorphine for bladder spasm. J Pain Symptom Manage 2003;25:1–2.
119. Picard PR, Tramer MR, McQuay HJ, et al. Analgesic efficacy of peripheral opioids (all except intra-articular): a qualitative systematic review of randomised controlled trials. Pain 1997;72:309–18.
120. Gupta A, Bodin L, Holmstrom B, et al. A systematic review of the peripheral analgesic effects of intraarticular morphine. Anesth Analg 2001;93:761–70.

Critical Monitoring Issues for Surgery Performed in a Non-hospital Setting

Samuel M. Galvagno, DO[a], Bhavani-Shankar Kodali, MD[b],*

KEYWORDS

- Out of operating room • Pulse oximetry
- Capnography • Monitoring • Anesthesia

Tremendous strides are evident in the nonsurgical interventional care delivered to patients outside of the operating rooms. In the past, both surgical and nonsurgical procedures were performed on sick patients primarily in the operating room (OR). However, recent technologic advances have facilitated the performance of a variety of procedures on complex patients outside of the OR. Many conditions that formerly required surgical intervention are now amenable to noninvasive treatment in interventional suites throughout the hospital.

Unfortunately, however, the physiological monitoring standards for patients undergoing these sophisticated procedures outside of the OR have not evolved concomitantly, and often they are below the standards of care being provided in the OR environment. The reasons for this disparity are that anesthesiologists are not involved in all aspects of care outside of the operating room (OOR), they may not be included in the initial planning stages of the OOR projects, and medical proceduralists are unfamiliar with the monitoring standards that are mandatory within the OR environment for similar procedures.

Improved standards of care in the OR have resulted in a remarkable decrease in morbidity and mortality in the last few decades, which is reflected by the significant decrease in the malpractice premiums of anesthesiologists. To ensure a safe environment for all patients, there is an urgent need to set forth and implement monitoring standards for the procedures performed outside of the ORs and to bring them into alignment with those of ORs. This is particularly necessary for patients with multiple comorbidities and will be increasingly important as non-OR procedures increase in complexity. Although definitive data are lacking, some findings have suggested that

This article originally appeared in *Anesthesiology Clinics of North America*, Volume 27, Issue 1.

[a] Johns Hopkins University School of Medicine, Baltimore, MD 21287, USA

[b] Department of Anesthesiology, Perioperative, and Pain Medicine, Brigham and Women's Hospital, Harvard Medical School, Boston, MA 0115, USA

* Corresponding author.

E-mail address: bkodali@partners.org (B-S. Kodali).

adverse events occurring during procedures performed outside of the OR environment have a higher severity of injury and may result from substandard care, including lack of adherence to minimum monitoring guidelines.[1] This review focuses on the physics, physiology, limitations, and recommendations for standard physiological monitors that should be used in the non-OR environment.

There are three important systems that should be monitored whenever procedures are performed in the OOR setting. They include circulation, ventilation, and oxygenation. Monitors to assess circulation are more often used and familiar to OOR personnel. OOR personnel are also familiar with pulse oximetry. However, OOR personnel are less familiar and often do not monitor ventilation and rely heavily on pulse oximetry as an indirect measure of ventilation. This is inadequate and unsafe. Anesthesiologists must impress upon their medical colleagues the difference between ventilation and oxygenation. Although apnea or hypoventilation usually precedes hypoxemia, the ensuing hypoxia is prevented easily if ventilation is directly monitored. Recognition of hypoventilation or apnea early will provide sufficient time to take corrective action before hypoxemia sets in. The value of capnography as a monitor of ventilation is highlighted in this review.

MONITORS
Pulse Oximetry

Many studies discovered significant knowledge deficits among clinicians regarding the limitations and interpretation of pulse oximetry results.[1-5] An understanding of pulse oximetry is obligatory for all proceduralists and nonanesthesiologists who provide non-OR care, because this technology is used as the principle means of assuring adequate oxygenation in a sedated or anesthetized patient.

Pulse oximetry relies on the spectral analysis of oxygenated and reduced hemoglobin and uses the principle of the Beer-Lambert law.[6-8] This law describes how the concentration of a substance in solution can be determined by transmitting a known intensity of light through a solution. With pulse oximetry, the oxygen saturation (SpO_2) is approximated by transmitting light of a specific wavelength across tissue and measuring its intensity on the other side. Red and near-infrared light readily penetrate tissue, whereas other wavelengths of light tend to be absorbed (**Fig. 1**).

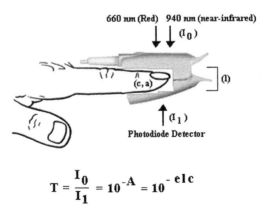

660 nm (Red)   940 nm (near-infrared)

$$T = \frac{I_0}{I_1} = 10^{-A} = 10^{-elc}$$

Fig. 1. Pulse oximetry: Application of the Beer-Lambert law. T, Transmittance; I_0, Intensity of incident light; I_1, Intensity of light after passing through material; A, Absorbance of smaple; l, Distance the light travels; a, Absorption coefficient of the absorber; e, Molar absorptivity of the absorber; c, Concentration of the absorbing species.

Light-emitting diodes are used to emit red light (660 nm) and near-infrared light (940 nm), because these two wavelengths have known absorption qualities when directed at hemoglobin (Hb). Specifically, 660-nm red light is absorbed by reduced Hb, whereas 940 nm is absorbed preferentially by oxygenated Hb. When these wavelengths are emitted through tissue and a vascular bed such as a finger, nostril, or earlobe, a photodiode detector on the opposite side measures the amount of light transmitted. The red/near-infrared ratio is calculated by the oximeter and compared with reference values for SpO_2 derived from healthy human subjects. The SpO_2 is further discriminated from venous blood or connective tissue by measuring the pulse-added component of the signal. This signal is comprised of alternating current, representing pulsatile arterial blood, and direct current, which corresponds to tissue, venous blood, and nonpulsatile arterial blood.[9] By canceling out the static components, the pulsatile component can be isolated and the SpO_2 estimated.

Pulse oximetry has several limitations. Nail polish and dark skin may cause a variable degree of interference; the physical obstruction to light transmittance appears to be related to darker skin pigmentation and dark-opaque nail polish.[10–12] In critically ill patients, a low signal-to-noise ratio may exist because of hypovolemia, peripheral vasoconstriction, or peripheral vascular disease.[13] Extra "noise" in the form of ambient light, deflection of light around and not through the vascular bed (optical shunt), and motion artifact may cause false readings.[14–16] Shivering is considered a common source of motion artifact, but normal pulse oximetry readings have been recorded in patients with tonic–clonic seizures.[17]

Dyshemoglobinemias represent a well-known cause of optical interference with pulse oximetry. Both carboxyhemoglobin (COHb) and methemoglobin (MetHb) absorb light within the red and near-infrared wavelength ranges used in pulse oximetry; standard pulse oximeters are unable to distinguish COHb and MetHb from normal oxyhemoglobin (O_2Hb). Hence, COHb will falsely absorb red light, and the pulse oximeter will display a falsely high saturation reading.[18] With MetHb, standard oximeters falsely detect a greater degree of absorption of both Hb and O_2Hb, increasing the absorbance ratio. When the absorbance ratio reaches 1, the calibrated saturation level approaches a plateau of approximately 85%.[19] Co-oximetry offers a multiwavelength analysis that takes into account the absorption of O_2Hb, MetHb, and COHb and should be used to determine an accurate saturation reading in cases in which these dyshemoglobins are suspected. Intravenous dyes such as methylene blue and indigo carmine cause reliable spurious decreases in oximetry readings.[20,21] Fetal hemoglobin, hyperbilirubinemia, and anemia have not been found to yield inaccurate oximetry readings in most cases.[22–24] Newer generations of pulse oximetry have overcome several of these limitations, particularly motion artifact and vasoconstriction. Some units measure carbon monoxide as well as MetHb levels. Measuring MetHb levels have become important with excessive use of benzocaine as local anesthesia for endoscopy procedures. Despite ongoing advances, it is not uncommon to obtain inconsistent waveforms and SpO_2 readings on hemodynamically unstable patients or patients with peripheral vascular disease. When pulse oximetry provides inadequate or unreliable measurements, reliance on monitors of ventilation and circulation becomes critical to ensuring patient well being during procedures.

Capnography

Over the last two decades, capnography has become a standard for monitoring in anesthesia practice.[25] The measurement of carbon dioxide (CO_2) in expired air directly indicates changes in the elimination of CO_2 from the lungs. Indirectly, it indicates changes in the production of CO_2 at the tissue level and in the delivery of CO_2 to the lungs by the circulatory system. Capnography is a noninvasive monitoring technique that allows fast and reliable insight into ventilation, circulation, and metabolism.[26] In the prehospital environment, it is used primarily for confirmation of successful endotracheal intubation, but it may also be a useful indicator of efficient ongoing cardiopulmonary resuscitation. Numerous national organizations, including the American Heart Association, now endorse capnography and capnographic methods for confirming endotracheal tube placement.[27] Despite these recommendations, capnography is not always widely available or consistently applied in the non-OR environment.[28]

Capnometry refers to the measurement and display of CO_2 on a digital or analog monitor. Maximum inspiratory and expiratory CO_2 concentrations during a respiratory cycle are displayed. Capnography refers to the graphic display of instantaneous CO_2 concentration (FCO_2) versus time or expired volume during a respiratory cycle (CO_2 waveform or capnogram). CO_2 waveforms are displayed as two types: FCO_2 versus expired volume (volume capnography) or against time (time capnography). Time capnography is the most common type used in clinical practice.

Infra-red (IR) spectrographs are the most compact and least expensive means to measure end-tidal CO_2 ($ETCO_2$). The wavelength of IR rays exceeds 1.0 millimicrons while the visible spectrum is between 0.4 and 0.8 mμ[29] The IR rays are absorbed by polyatomic gases such as nitrous oxide, CO_2, and water vapor. CO_2 selectively absorbs specific wavelengths (4.3 millimicrons) of IR light (**Fig. 2**). Because the amount of light absorbed is proportional to the concentration of the absorbing molecules, the concentration of a gas can be determined by comparing the measured absorbance with the absorbance of a known standard. The CO_2 concentration measured by the monitor is usually expressed as partial pressure in millimeters of mercury, although some units display percentage CO_2, obtained by dividing the partial pressure of CO_2 by the atmospheric pressure. Other techniques used to measure $ETCO_2$ include Raman spectrography, molecular correlation spectography, mass spectography, and photoacoustic spectography. Infrared technology is cheaper compared with others, and hence is the method of choice used in most capnographs.

A standard terminology for capnography has been adapted.[30] A time capnogram can be divided into inspiratory (phase 0) and expiratory segments (**Fig. 3**). The expiratory segment, similar to a single breath nitrogen curve or single breath CO_2 curve, is divided into three phases (phases I, II, and III). The angle between phase II and phase III is the alpha angle. Alpha angle is an indirect measure of ventilation–perfusion (V/Q) status of the lung. The nearly 90° angle between phase III and the descending limb is the beta angle. Increases in beta angle may indicate presence of rebreathing. The maximal value of expired CO_2 at the end of the expiration is known as end-tidal CO_2 ($ETCO_2$). It can be expressed as percentage CO_2 or, more commonly, as partial

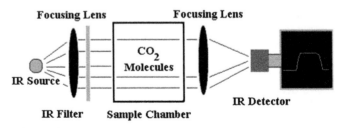

Fig. 2. IR spectrography.

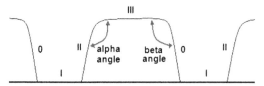

Fig. 3. Current terminology for components of a time capnogram.

pressure in millimeters of mercury ($PETCO_2$). Some causes of increased or decreased $ETCO_2$ are shown in **Box 1**.

Under normal circumstances, the $PETCO_2$ is lower than arterial PCO_2 ($PaCO_2$) by 2 to 5 mm Hg, in adults.[31–34] The PCO_2 gradient is caused by the V/Q mismatch in the lungs as a result of temporal, spatial, and alveolar mixing defects. The arterial-to-end-tidal (a-ET) PCO_2/$PaCO_2$ fraction is a measure of alveolar dead space, and changes in alveolar dead space correlate well with changes in (a-ET) PCO_2.[30] An increase in (a-ET) PCO_2 suggests an increase in dead space ventilation; hence, (a-ET) PCO_2 can provide an indirect estimate of V/Q mismatching of the lung. End-tidal PCO_2 can be used to estimate $PaCO_2$ if there are no abrupt changes in cardiac output or ventilation. However, if there is hemodynamic instability, (a-ET) PCO_2 can vary with varying perfusion to lungs. This changes the ventilation–perfusion relationship, and thereby results in variations in alveolar dead space. Under these circumstances, $PETCO_2$ may not reliably estimate $PaCO_2$.

For a given ventilation, a reduction in cardiac output and pulmonary blood flow results in a decrease in PETCO2 and an increase in (a-ET) PCO_2. Increases in cardiac output and pulmonary blood flow result in better perfusion of the alveoli and an increase in $PETCO_2$.[35] The decrease in (a-ET) PCO_2 is caused by an increase in the alveolar CO_2 suggesting better excretion of CO_2 into the lungs. The improved CO_2 excretion is caused by better perfusion of upper parts of the lung. There is an inverse

---

Box 1
Causes of increased or decreased CO_2

Causes of Increased CO_2

Hypoventilation

Hyperthyroidism/Thyroid Storm

Malignant Hyperthermia

Fever/Sepsis

Rebreathing

Other Hypermetabolic States

Causes of Decreased CO_2

Hyperventilation

Hypothermia

Venous Air Embolism

Pulmonary Embolism

Decreased Cardiac Output

Hypoperfusion

linear correlation between pulmonary artery pressure and (a-ET) PCO_2.[36] Thus, under conditions of constant lung ventilation, $PETCO_2$ monitoring can be used as a monitor of pulmonary blood flow. Cardiac output and $PETCO_2$ studies have shown good correlation between each other. An $ETCO_2$ of 32 mm Hg and 36 mm Hg correlated with a cardiac output 4 L and 5 L, respectively, in intubated and ventilated subjects.

Because of varying (a-ET) PCO_2 in some patients, transcutaneous monitoring of PCO_2 has been used as an alternative to $ETCO_2$ monitoring. In one study of 17 elderly patients, transcutaneous monitoring of PCO_2 provided a more accurate estimation of arterial CO_2 partial pressure than $PETCO_2$ monitoring.[37] At the time of this writing, transcutaneous PCO_2 monitoring is not yet widely available, and the role of this modality for monitoring in the OOR environment has yet to be defined.

End-tidal PCO_2 measurements can also be easily performed in nonintubated spontaneously breathing patients receiving oxygen. However, the resulting waveforms and $PETCO_2$ measurements can be distorted by a dilution effect of air or oxygen resulting in decreased $PETCO_2$ readings. Several varieties of mask and sampling devices are available on the market that provide measurements close to those obtained in intubated patients. Even if the measurements are not quantitatively accurate, they can be considered as baseline measurements/waveforms, and any deviations from baseline during sedation should indicate respiratory depression (see **Figs. 3** and **4**, www. capnography.com, sedation section).

Blood Pressure Measurement

Blood pressure in OOR locations is commonly measured with noninvasive oscillometric devices. An electronic pressure transducer detects oscillating blood flow as the

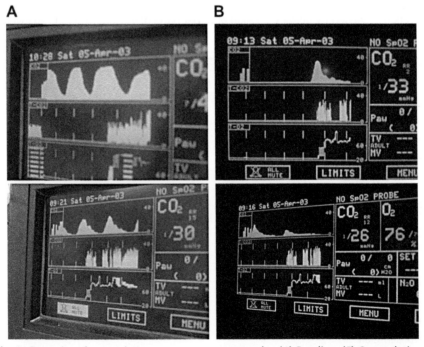

Fig. 4. Examples of oversedation as seen on capnography. (*A*) Baseline. (*B*) Oversedation.

cuff is deflated. Assuming the upper extremity is used, the compressed brachial artery oscillates as restricted blood flows through it and the systolic, diastolic, and mean pressures are determined. An in-depth discussion of invasive intra-arterial techniques is beyond the scope of this article; for further information, an excellent review by Polanco and Pinsky is available.[38]

Electrocardiography

Both transmural and subendocardial ischemia can be detected when electrocardiography (ECG) leads are properly positioned.[39] Lead V_5, the precordial lead originally described in Kaplan and King's classic report on intraoperative ischemia, has been validated and found to detect up to 75% of ischemic changes seen in all 12 leads.[40,41] The combination of leads II, V_2, V_3, V_4, and V_5, has a sensitivity of 100% for detecting intraoperative ischemia.[39] The reader is directed to an exceptional review on perioperative electrocardiography previously published in *Anesthesiology Clinics*.[42]

Temperature Monitoring

Perioperative hypothermia increases the incidence of adverse myocardial outcomes, increases blood loss, and increases wound infection.[43–45] Mild hypothermia also changes the kinetics of various anesthetics and may delay postoperative recovery.[45] Intraoperative hypothermia usually develops in three phases. The first phase is caused by redistribution of heat from the core thermal compartment to the outer shell of the body. A slower, linear reduction in the core temperature follows and may last several hours.[45] In the last phase, the core temperature plateaus and may remain unchanged throughout the remainder of the perioperative period as thermoregulatory control is impaired during general or regional anesthesia. Numerous temperature monitoring devices are available, but it is the site of temperature monitoring rather than the type of temperature probe that is most important. Core temperature can be estimated from accessible sites such as the nasopharynx, bladder, esophageal, or rectal sites.[45] Temperature monitoring has become a standard of care, and anesthesiologists are expected to be proactive in maintaining normothermia and preventing temperature derangements throughout the perioperative period. Most of the OOR environments are kept at lower temperatures to protect the expensive equipment. Therefore, it is essential that temperature monitoring is an integral part of the monitoring systems in OOR.

Spontaneous Electroencephalographic Activity Monitors

Depth of anesthesia monitoring with the bispectral index monitor (BIS) has been shown to reduce, but not eliminate, the incidence of awareness under anesthesia.[46] In the neurocritical care setting, BIS monitoring has been shown to provide a more objective means of sedation assessment that may lead to a decrease in overall rates of propofol administration and fewer incidences of oversedation.[47] A recent Cochrane review concluded that anesthesia guided by BIS within the recommended range (40 to 60) could improve anesthetic delivery and postoperative recovery from relatively deep anesthesia while reducing the incidence of intraoperative recall in surgical patients at a high risk for awareness.[48] The Patient State Index (PSI) is another monitor for awareness that has not been studied as thoroughly as the BIS, but has been shown to provide indications that correlate with unconsciousness.[49] For a detailed review of the current state of monitors for preventing intraoperative awareness, the reader is directed to the American Society of Anesthesiologists' (ASA's) 2006 Practice Advisory.[50]

CONSIDERATIONS FOR MONITORING IN OUT-OF-OR ENVIRONMENTS
The Magnetic Resonance Imaging Suite

Magnetic resonance imaging (MRI) poses a profound risk to patients with implanted ferromagnetic material because the high magnetic field may dislodge pacemakers, implants, cardiac valves, or other prostheses. Before entering the MRI suite, all ferromagnetic items need to be removed from the care provider's possession to prevent injury; an MRI-compatible anesthesia machine and equipment are compulsory.[51] The intense radiofrequency may cause surface heating on the patient's body, and the lead wires from the ECG also pose a potential burn hazard.[52] The ECG monitor is subject to considerable artifact from the background static magnetic field and radiofrequency impulses as well as the electronics within the device that create magnetic fields.[53] Modern devices minimize these limitations and advances in ECG monitoring in the MRI suite continue. Blood pressure monitoring by the oscillometric method is most commonly used and provides reliable readings. Pulse oximetry may be difficult in the MRI suite because the signal may become degraded as a result of currents in the oximetry cable and a decreased signal-to-noise ratio.[54] A decrease in the phase II slope of the capnogram may be observed because of a long circuit pathway. Remote monitoring via a closed-circuit monitor—preferably with zoom lens magnification capability—may be necessary. Several MRI-compatible monitors measure cardiovascular, ventilatory (capnography), and oxygenation (pulse oximetry) reliably, and, therefore, all patients undergoing MRI can be monitored as they would be in the OR.

Computed Tomography

An anesthetized patient in the computed tomography (CT) scanner presents logistical problems similar to those encountered in the MRI suite; however, the impact on interference with standard monitors is not as profound. Blood pressure should be monitored at relatively short intervals because radiocontrast media reactions may lead to a precipitous loss of systemic vascular resistance. Standard monitors such as the ECG, temperature probe, pulse oximetry, and capnography should be used. As with procedures done in the MRI suite and elsewhere, remote monitoring may be required. Frequently, apnea is requested during fluoroscopy, and capnography is essential to serve as a reminder to start the ventilator if forgotten inadvertently.

Electroconvulsive Therapy

Electroconvulsive therapy (ECT) is used for treatment of severe psychiatric disorders as well as depression, complex regional pain syndrome, and chronic pain.[55] ECT involves provocation of a generalized epileptic seizure by electrical stimulation of the brain. The procedure usually is preformed under general anesthesia with muscle relaxation. Excessive alterations in heart rate, blood pressure, and cardiac functions are prevented by anticholinergic and antihypertensive agents; hence, blood pressure and ECG monitoring is mandatory.[56] Train-of-four monitoring for neuromuscular blockade and BIS monitoring should also be considered. Capnography is essential for safe and effective anesthetic management of patients undergoing ECT, especially patients with intracranial disorders or coronary artery disease.[57]

The Endoscopy Suite

Most endoscopic procedures are performed in an OOR environment, and in many cases, these procedures may be accomplished with moderate or deep sedation. Capnography should be used because significant delays in detecting respiratory compromise have been shown in its absence.[58] In addition to blood pressure and ECG monitoring, pulse oximetry and capnography should be considered standard monitors to ensure adequate ventilation and oxygenation during endoscopic procedures, whether they be performed under general anesthesia or varying degrees of sedation.[59] The American Society of Gastrointestinal Endoscopy and the British Society of Gastroenterology issue guidelines periodically to impress upon practitioners the need to be proactive in detecting and eliminating hypoxia during gastrointestinal procedures.

Interventional Angiography

ECG, blood pressure, pulse oximetry, and capnography are standard monitors for procedures in interventional angiography. In addition, intracranial pressure monitoring (ICP) and invasive arterial blood pressure monitoring are frequently used. In some instances, central venous pressure monitoring and monitoring of evoked potentials may be necessary. In recent years, the endovascular treatment of diseases of intracranial and spinal vessels has become widely accepted; invasive monitoring is frequently required based on the usual underlying pathophysiology and severity of these disorders.[60]

Controversies in monitoring

Numerous investigators have focused in the ability of monitors to prevent morbidity and mortality. In a well-known randomized, controlled trial by Watkinson and colleagues,[61] the investigators concluded that mandated electronic vital signs monitoring in high-risk medical and surgical patients had no effect on adverse events or mortality. Although this study had numerous limitations that may have led to type II error, the "number needed to monitor" to alter outcomes was estimated to be large.[61] In a systematic review of randomized, controlled trials examining the role of pulse oximetry, there was no evidence of a significant difference between groups regarding duration of postoperative mechanical ventilation, duration of intensive care unit stay, or postoperative complications; the investigators were unable to find reliable evidence that pulse oximetry affects the outcome of anesthesia.[62] Moller's landmark studies in 1993, based on a design that was similar to both a randomized, controlled trial and a cluster randomized trial that included 20,802 patients, concluded that pulse oximetry did not have a significant impact on mortality or hospital stay.[63–65] In a review of clinical trials on monitoring, the authors acknowledge that pulse oximetry may enable clinicians to detect desaturation episodes more readily and that this technology may be beneficial, but to prevent one adverse event, a large number of patients must be monitored.[66] The findings of these and other related studies were summarized in a Cochrane review that concluded that the value of perioperative monitoring with pulse oximetry is unproven.[67]

Earlier studies, including a closed claims analysis, suggested that pulse oximetry was an invaluable modality for preventing adverse outcomes in anesthesia, and that improvements in monitoring—specifically pulse oximetry—may have helped reduce serious mishaps over the last several decades by at least 35%.[68] Two additional studies suggested that monitoring with pulse oximetry facilitates early detection of arterial hypoxemia, allowing earlier and potentially life-saving treatment.[65,69] Oversedation with ensuing respiratory depression is an important contributor to adverse events that have occurred under monitored anesthesia care, and appropriate use of monitoring has been cited as a crucial preventative measure that often is neglected.[70] Studies based on analyses of closed claims data suggest that better monitoring may lead to earlier correction of potentially harmful perioperative events.[71,72]

Despite numerous national guidelines and recommendations, there seems to be a paucity of data to support the use of monitors in preventing mortality outside of the OR. In 2006, Watkinson and colleagues[61] studied 402 heterogeneous high-risk medical and surgical ward patients, and failed to demonstrate that monitoring heart rate, noninvasive blood pressure, oxygen saturation, respiratory rate by impedance pneumography, and skin temperature could predict or identify adverse outcomes. Similarly, when a medical emergency team was tasked with closely following vital signs in an effort to rapidly recognize critical threshold patterns suggestive of potential adverse events, no benefit was found.[73] Although each of these studies had significant limitations, they helped promulgate the idea that mandatory monitoring, even with a high incidence of abnormal vital signs, does not confer a mortality benefit. Nevertheless, other investigators determined that improved monitoring might have prevented a significant number of adverse outcomes identified in the ASA closed claims database.[74]

Initial studies using capnography as a supplement during procedures requiring sedation suggested that this practice might serve as an early warning mechanism for impending respiratory embarrassment.[75,76] Capnography may have an advantage over pulse oximetry because capnography is a better measure of ventilation. With capnography, providers are able to institute early stimulation for nonbreathing patients, thereby preventing arterial oxygen desaturation. Lightdale and colleagues[77] found that microstream capnography significantly prevented arterial oxygen desaturation in children undergoing sedation for procedures. This was an important finding because most of the calamitous events during sedation occur secondarily to hypoventilation and respiratory failure.[78]

The zone between sedation and anesthesia is very narrow. When the patient drifts away from conscious sedation to a state in which there is no response to verbal commands or sensory stimuli, he approaches general anesthesia. The width of this safety zone depends on the physical condition of the patient, amount of sedatives used, potency of medications, and stimulation arising from the procedure. When the stimulation suddenly ceases, this can induce a relative excess of sedation leading to hypoventilation or apnea. If not readily detected and corrected, this can culminate in hypoxemia. Sometimes, visual observation of patient is not possible, either because of the type of procedure or dark rooms that are necessary for good visualization of LCD screens by the interventionists performing noninvasive procedures. Therefore, it is likely that every patient being given so-called "conscious sedation," at some time or the other during the course of the sedation procedure, will drift into a state of deep sedation or general anesthesia. The duration of this depends on the factors enumerated above. Hence, it can be logically argued that any patient receiving sedation also qualifies for ASA standards of monitoring and should have their circulatory, ventilatory, and oxygenation status monitored in standard fashion. Ironically, administration of supplementary oxygen to the patients compounds the problem further. The goal of supplemental oxygen is to increase oxygen reserves, thereby delaying or preventing the onset of hypoxia. It has been shown that super oxygenated patients desaturate only after prolonged apnea.[79,80] This negates the use of pulse oximetry as an early warning monitoring device for respiratory depression, which is concerning in light of the fact that the majority of sedation providers rarely recognize respiratory depression in sedated patients who do not become hypoxic.[81] In one study, the treating physicians blinded to capnography could not identify apneic episodes during sedation procedures.[82] In the same study, absolute $ETCO_2$ change of greater than 10 mm Hg identified nine of 25 patients who experienced hypoxia (36% sensitive) (95% confidence interval [CI], 18% to 57%) and 68% specific (95% CI, 57% to

77%); positive predictive value (PPV), 32%; negative predictive value (NPPV), 67%. An absolute $ETCO_2$ change from baseline of greater than 10% would have identified 18 of the 25 patients before hypoxia developed (sensitivity, 72% [95% CI, 59% to 93%]; specificity, 47% [95% CI, 36% to 58%]; PPV, 37%; NPV, 80%).

RECOMMENDATIONS

Although data to support a mortality benefit appear to be lacking, numerous organizations, including the ASA, strongly endorse monitoring in OOR environments.[83,84] A letter in the *British Medical Journal* was concerned about the relatively higher death rate of 1 in 2000 from upper gastrointestinal endoscopy, which is usually performed under sedation or local anesthesia, or both,[85] compared with the overall morality solely attributable to anesthesia, which is 1 in 185,000 or higher. The OR environment has become safer because of stringent monitoring standards. There is an urgent need to take proactive measures and follow a set of standard guidelines to enhance the safety of patients undergoing OOR procedures. It is only a matter of time before medico-legal scenarios will shift to OOR locations, where more patients will be cared for, and inadequate monitoring may contribute to morbidity and mortality. For OOR anesthetizing locations, the ASA recommends that the Standards for Basic Anesthetic Monitoring (**Table 1**) be followed.[86]

In a busy hospital practice, it is not uncommon to hear "code blue" being called from OOR locations. The majority of these emergencies are ventilation-related incidents that occur during procedural sedation performed by nonanesthesiologists. If anesthesiologists provide sedation, capnography typically is used in addition to other monitors, as recommended by ASA. When sedation is administered by nonanesthesia personnel, we strongly recommend that ventilation be monitored during all procedures (**Table 2**). There is ongoing educational process in our institution to train nonanesthesia personnel in the value of capnography as a ventilation monitor. At the moment, capnography seems to be the best available device for ventilatory monitoring. Hence, it is the onus of physicians overseeing sedation procedures to encourage the monitoring ventilation to increase the safety of the patients under their care.

Table 1	
Standards for basic anesthetic monitoring	
Parameter	**Methods**
Equipment	Anesthesia equipment, machine should be set up in standard format identical to OR to minimize unfamiliarity to the anesthesiologists.
Oxygenation	Inspired gas oxygen analyzer pulse oximetry (with audible tone). Illumination to assess the patient's color.
Ventilation	$PETCO_2$ monitoring: Capnography with audible CO_2 alarm to detect correct placement of endotracheal tube. Use of a device capable of detecting disconnection of the components of the breathing system. Detection of hypoventilation.
Circulation	Continuous electrocardiogram blood pressure and heart rate determination no less than every 5 minutes. Assessment by at least one of the following: palpation of a pulse, intra-arterial tracing of blood pressure, ultrasound peripheral pulse monitoring, pulse plethysmography, or oximetry.
Body Temperature	Indicated when clinical significant changes in body temperature are intended, anticipated, or suspected.

| Table 2 |
| Recommended monitoring for procedural sedation |

Parameter	Methods
Training	Physicians must understand the value of monitoring and undergo procedural sedation course.
Establishment of protocols	All the OOR sites should have uniform protocols so that their implementation is easy and uniform across all sites.
Oxygenation	Pulse oximetry (with audible tone). Illumination to assess the patient's color.
Ventilation	PETCO$_2$ monitoring: Capnography with audible CO$_2$ alarm to detect hypoventilation and apnea.
Circulation	Continuous electrocardiogram. Blood pressure and heart rate determination no less than every 5 minutes.
Body Temperature	Indicated when clinical significant changes in body temperature are expected during long noninvasive procedures.
Review protocols	Periodic review of problems encountered and appropriate amendments made to protocols to ensure that the problems do not recur.

SUMMARY

Monitoring standards in OOR locations should not differ from those in the OR. Because of extraordinary developments in medical, surgical, and radiologic techniques, sicker patients are being cared for outside of traditional ORs. It is essential that we keep pace with these evolving changes and make improvements needed to provide the same standard of monitoring care outside of the OR as we rely on in the ORs. Furthermore, some of the OOR locations are remote from main operating locations, and it may take considerable time to respond to any emergencies and codes that may arise in these locations. Although the true rate of complications from anesthesia in the OOR environment is currently unknown, we should not wait to implement standards for monitoring until disasters occur. There is no need to reinvent the wheel to determine the need for vigilant monitoring in OOR settings. Anesthesiologists have evolved a robust system of monitoring standards based on decades of experience in OR environments. Every OOR location should be thoroughly evaluated with monitoring standards implemented. These standards should be periodically reviewed to avert morbidity.

REFERENCES

1. Robbertze R, Posner K, Domino K. Closed claims review of anesthesia for procedures outside the operating room. Curr Opin Anaesthesiol 2006;19:436–42.
2. Sinex J. Pulse oximetry: principles and limitations. Am J Emerg Med 1999;17:59–67.
3. Elliott M, Tate R, Page K. Do clinicians know how to use pulse oximetry? A literature review and clinical implications. Aust Crit Care 2006;19:139–44.
4. Rodriguez L, Kotin N, Lowenthal D, et al. A study of pediatric house staff's knowledge of pulse oximetry. Pediatrics 1994;93:810–3.
5. Stoneham M, Saville G, Wilson I. Knowledge about pulse oximetry among medical and nursing staff. Lancet 1994;344:1339–42.

6. Kelleher J. Pulse oximetry. J Clin Monit 1989;5:37–62.
7. Tremper K, Barker S. Pulse oximetry. Anesthesiology 1989;70:98–108.
8. Salyer J. Neonatal and pediatric pulse oximetry. Respir Care 2003;48:386–96.
9. Wukitsch M, Petterson M, Tobler DR, et al. Pulse oximetry: analysis of theory, technology, and practice. J Clin Monit 1988;4:290–301.
10. Volgyesi G, Spahr-Schopfer I. Does skin pigmentation affect the accuracy of pulse oximetry? An in vitro study. Anesthesiology 1991;75:A406.
11. Cote C, Goldsteing E, Fuchsman W, et al. The effect of nail polish on pulse oximetry. Anesth Analg 1988;67:683–6.
12. Ries A, Prewitt L, Johnson J. Skin color and ear oximetry. Chest 1989;96:287–90.
13. Severinghaus J, Spellman M. Pulse oximeter failure thresholds in hypotension and vasoconstriction. Anesthesiology 1990;73:532–7.
14. Hanowell L, Eisele JH, Downs D. Ambient light affects pulse oximeters. Anesthesiology 1987;67:864–5.
15. Costarino A, Davis D, Keon T. Falsely normal saturation reading with the pulse oximeter. Anesthesiology 1987;67:830–1.
16. Severinghaus JW, Kelleher JF. Recent developments in pulse oximetry. Anesthesiology 1992;76(6):1018–38.
17. James M, Marshall H, Carew-McColl M. Pulse oximetry during apparent tonic-clonic seizures. Lancet 1991;337:394–5.
18. Buckley R, Aks S, Eshom J, et al. The pulse oximetry gap in carbon monoxide intoxication. Ann Emerg Med 1994;24:252–5.
19. Barker S, Tremper KK, Hyatt J. Effects of methemoglobinemia on pulse oximetry and mixed venous oximetry. Anesthesiology 1989;70:112–7.
20. Kessler M, Eide T, Humayan B, et al. Spurious pulse oximeter desaturation with methylene blue injection. Anesthesiology 1986;65:435–6.
21. Scheller M, Unger R, Kelner M. Effects of intravenously administered dyes on pulse oximetry readings. Anesthesiology 1986;65:550–2.
22. Severinghaus J, Koh S. Effect of anemia on pulse oximeter accuracy at low saturation. J Clin Monit 1990;85–8.
23. Harris A, Sendak M, Donham R, et al. Absorption characteristics of human fetal hemoglobin at wavelengths used in pulse oximetry. J Clin Monit 1988;4:175–7.
24. Ramanathan R, Durand M, Larrazabal C. Pulse oximetry in very low birth weight infants with acute and chronic disease. Pediatrics 1987;79(4):612–7.
25. Kodali B, Moseley H, Kumar A, et al. Capnography and anaesthesia: review article. Can J Anaesth 1992;39:617–32.
26. Kupnik D, Skok P. Capnometry in the prehospital setting: are we using its potential? J Emerg Med 2007;24:614–7.
27. American Heart Association. 2005 American heart association guidelines for cardiopulmonary resuscitation and emergency cardiovascular care. Part 7.1: adjuncts for airway control and ventilation. Circulation 2005;112:IV-51–7.
28. Deiorio M. Continuous end-tidal carbon dioxide monitoring for confirmation of endotracheal tube placement is neither widely available nor consistently applied by emergency physicians. J Emerg Med 2005;22:490–3.
29. Colman Y, Krauss B. Microstream capnography technology: a new approach to an old problem. J Clin Monit 1999;15.
30. Kodali B, Kumar A, Moseley H, et al. Terminology and the current limitations of time capnography: A brief review. J Clin Monit 1995;11:175–82.
31. Nunn J, Hill D. Respiratory dead space and arterial to end-tidal CO_2 tension difference in anesthetized man. J Appl Phys 1960;15:383–9.

32. Fletcher R, Jonson B. Deadspace and the single breath test carbon dioxide during anaesthesia and artificial ventilation. Br J Anaesth 1984;56:109–19.

33. Kodali B, Moseley H, Kumar Y, et al. Arterial to end-tidal carbon dioxide tension difference during Caesarean section anaesthesia. Anaesthesia 1986;41: 698–702.

34. Fletcher R, Jonson B, Cumming G, et al. The concept of dead space with special reference to the single breath test for carbon dioxide. Br J Anaesth 1981;53: 77–88.

35. Leigh M, Jones J, Motley H. The expired carbon dioxide as a continuous guide of the pulmonary and circulatory systems during anesthesia and surgery. J Thorac Cardiovasc Surg 1961;41:597–610.

36. Askrog V. Changes in (a-A) CO2 difference and pulmonary artery pressure in anesthetized man. J Appl Phys 1966;21:1299–305.

37. Casati A, Squicciarini G, Malagutti G, et al. Transcutaneous monitoring of partial pressure of carbon dioxide in the elderly patient: a prospective, clinical comparison with end-tidal monitoring. J Clin Anesth 2006;18:436–40.

38. Polanco P, Pinsky M. Practical issues of hemodynamic monitoring at the bedside. Surg Clin North Am 2006;86:1431–56.

39. Fuchs R, Achuff S, Grunwald L, et al. Electrocardiographic localization of coronary artery narrowings: studies during myocardial ischemia and infarction in patients with one-vessel disease. Circulation 1982;66:1168–76.

40. Kaplan J, King S. The precordial electrocardiographic lead (V5) in patients who have coronary-artery disease. Anesthesiology 1976;45:570–4.

41. London M, Hollenberg M, Wong W, et al. Intraoperative myocardial ischemia: localization by continuous 12-lead electrocardiography. Anesthesiology 1988; 69:232–41.

42. John A, Fleisher L. Electrocardiography: the ECG. Anesthesiol Clin 2006;24: 697–715.

43. Kurz A, Sessler D, Lenhardt R. Perioperative normothermia to reduce the incidence of surgical-wound infection and shorten hospitalization. Study of wound infection and temperature group. N Engl J Med 1996;334:1209–15.

44. Pestel GJ, Kurz A. Hypothermia—it's more than a toy. Curr Opin Anaesthesiol 2005;18(2):151–6.

45. Insler S, Sessler D. Perioperative thermoregulation and temperature monitoring. Anesthesiol Clin 2006;24:823–37.

46. Bruhn J, Myles P, Sneyd R, et al. Depth of anaesthesia monitoring: what's available, what's validated and what's next? Br J Anaesth 2006;97:85–94.

47. Olson D, Cheek D, Morgenlander J. The impact of bispectral index monitoring on rates of propofol administration. AACN clinical issues: advanced practice in acute & critical care. Biol Med 2004;1:63–73.

48. Punjasawadwong Y, Boonjeungmonkol N, Phongchiewboon A. Bispectral index for improving anaesthetic delivery and postoperative recovery. Cochrane Database Syst Rev 2007;4:CD003843.

49. Chen X, Tang J, White P, et al. A comparison of patient state index and bispectral index values during the perioperative period. Anesth Analg 2002;95: 1669–74.

50. Apfelbaum J, Arens J, Cole D, et al. for the American Society of Anesthesiologists Task Force on Intraoperative Awareness. Practice advisory for intraoperative awareness and brain function monitoring. Anesthesiology 2006;104:847–64.

51. Deckert D, Zecha-Stallinger A, Haas T, et al. Anesthesia outside the core operating area. Anaesthesist 2007;56:1028–30, 32–7.

52. Rejger V, Cohn B, Vielvoye G, et al. A simple anaesthetic and monitoring system for magnetic resonance imaging. Eur J Anaesthesiol 1989;6:373–8.
53. Patterson S, Chesney J. Anesthetic management for magnetic resonance imaging: problems and solutions. Anesth Analg 1992;74(1):121–8.
54. Peden CJ, Menon DK, Hall AS, et al. Magnetic resonance for the anaesthetist. Anesthesia 1992;47(6):508–17.
55. Grundmann U, Oest M. Anaesthesiological aspects of electroconvulsive therapy. Anaesthesist 2007;56:202–4, 6–11.
56. Saito S. Anesthesia management for electroconvulsive therapy: hemodynamic and respiratory management. J Anesth 2005;19:142–9.
57. Saito S, Kadoi Y, Nihishara F, et al. End-tidal carbon dioxide monitoring stabilized hemodynamic changes during ECT. J ECT 2003;19:26–30.
58. Pino R. The nature of anesthesia and procedural sedation outside of the operating room. Curr Opin Anaesthesiol 2007;20:347–51.
59. Melloni C. Anesthesia and sedation outside the operating room: how to prevent risk and maintain good quality. Curr Opin Anaesthesiol 2007;20:513–9.
60. Preiss H, Reinartz J, Lowens S, et al. Anesthesiological management of neuroendovascular interventions. Anaesthesist 2006;55:679–92.
61. Watkinson P, Barber V, Price J, et al. A randomised controlled trial of the effect of continuous electronic physiological monitoring on the adverse event rate in high risk medical and surgical patients. Anesthesia 2006;61:1031–9.
62. Pedersen T, Moller AM, Pedersen BD. Pulse oximetry for perioperative monitoring: systematic review of randomized, controlled trials. Anesth Analg 2003; 96(2):426–31.
63. Moller J, Johannessen N, Espersen K, et al. Randomized evaluation of pulse oximetry in 20,802 patients: II. Perioperative events and postoperative complications. Anesthesiology 1993;78:445–53.
64. Moller J, Pedersen T, Rasmussen L, et al. Randomized evaluation of pulse oximetry in 20,802 patients: I. Design, demography, pulse oximetry failure rate, and overall complication rate. Anesthesiology 1993;78:436–44.
65. Moller J, Wittrup M, Johansen S. Hypoxemia in the postanesthesia care unit: an observer study. Anesthesiology 1990;73:890–5.
66. Young D, Griffiths J. Clinical trials of monitoring in anaesthesia, critical care and acute ward care: a review. Br J Anaesth 2006;97:39–45.
67. Pedersen T, Pedersen B, Moller A. Pulse oximetry for Perioperative monitoring. Cochrane Database Syst Rev 2003;3:CD002013.
68. Tinker J, Dull D, Caplan R, et al. Role of monitoring devices in prevention of anesthetic mishaps: a closed claims analysis. Anesthesiology 1989;71:541–6.
69. Cote CJ, Rolf N, Liu LM, et al. A single-blind study of combined pulse oximetry and capnography in children. Anesthesiology 1991;74(6):980–7.
70. Bhananker S, Posner K, Cheney F, et al. Injury and liability associated with monitored anesthesia care: a closed claims analysis. Anesthesiology 2006;104: 228–34.
71. Cooper J, Cullen D, Nemeskal R, et al. Effects of information feedback and pulse oximetry on the incidence of anesthesia complications. Anesthesiology 1987;67: 686–94.
72. Cooper J, Newbower R, Kitz R. An analysis of major errors and equipment failures in anesthesia management: considerations for prevention and detection. Anesthesiology 1984;60:34–42.
73. Hillman K, Chen J, Cretikos M, et al. Introduction of the medical emergency team (MET) system: a cluster-randomized controlled trial. Lancet 2005;365:2091–7.

74. Caplan R, Posner K, Ward R, et al. Adverse respiratory events in anesthesia: a closed claims analysis. Anesthesiology 1990;72:828–33.
75. Soto R, Fu E, Vila H, et al. Capnography accurately detects apnea during monitored anesthesia care. Anesth Analg 2004;99:379–82.
76. Vargo J, Zuccaro G, Dumot J, et al. Automated graphic assessment of respiratory activity is superior to pulse oximetry and visual assessment for the detection of early respiratory depression during therapeutic upper endoscopy. Gastrointest Endosc 2002;55:826–31.
77. Lightdale J, Goldmann D, Feldman H, et al. Microstream capnography improves patient monitoring during moderate sedation: a randomized, controlled trial. Pediatrics 2006;117:e1170–80.
78. Cote C, Notterman D, Karl H. Adverse sedation events in pediatrics: a critical incident analysis of contributing factors. Pediatrics 2000;105:805–14.
79. Jense HG, Dubin SA, Silverstein PI, et al. Effect of obesity on safe duration of apnea in anesthetized humans. Anesth Analg 1991;72:89–93.
80. Patel R, Lenczyk M, Hannallah RS, et al. Age and the onset of desaturation in apnoeic children. Can J Anaesth 1994;41:771–4.
81. Deitch K, Chudnofsky CR, Dominici P. The utility of supplemental oxygen during emergency department procedural sedation and analgesia with midozolam and fentanyl: a randomized, controlled trial. Ann Emerg Med 2007;49:1–8.
82. Deitch K, Chudnofsky CR, Dominici P. The utility of supplemental oxygen during emergency department procedural sedation with propofol: a randomized, controlled trial. Ann Emerg Med 2008;52:1–8.
83. The American Society of Anesthesiologists. Guidelines for nonoperating room anesthetizing locations. 2003. Avaliable at: http://www.asahq.org/publications AndServices/standards/14.pdf. 2003. Accessed June 23, 2008.
84. Cote C, Wilson S, Sedation and the Workgroup on Sedation. Guidelines for monitoring and management of pediatric patients during and after sedation for diagnostic and therapeutic procedures. Pediatrics 2006;118:2587–602.
85. Appaddurai IR, Delicta RJ, Carey PD, et al. Monitoring during endoscopy. BMJ 1995;311(7002):452.
86. The American Society of Anesthesiologists. Standards for basic anesthetic monitoring. 2005. Avaliable at: http://www.asahq.org/publicationsAndServices/ standards/02.pdf. 2005. Accessed June 23, 2008.

Anesthesia for Gastrointestinal Endoscopic Procedures

Daniel T. Goulson, MD*, Regina Y. Fragneto, MD

KEYWORDS

- Anesthesia • Sedation
- Esophagogastroduodenoscopy • Colonoscopy
- Endoscopic retrograde cholangiopancreatography
- Endoscopic ultrasonography

The provision of sedation and analgesia always has been a critical component of performing endoscopic procedures on the gastrointestinal (GI) tract. The procedures create some pain and discomfort and are associated with anxiety for the patient. Of course, comfort is paramount, but patient cooperation also is critical to the success of the examination. In the early days of endoscopy, it was routine practice for the sedation and analgesia to be provided by the endoscopist, who ordered a benzodiazepine, such as diazepam, and an opioid, such as meperidine, that were administered by a nurse. Monitoring was provided by periodic visual observation by the physician and/or the nurse. The administration of supplemental oxygen was inconsistent.

In the current environment, things are changing. The demand for endoscopy, especially screening colonoscopies, has increased dramatically. More stimulating and complex procedures that can be accomplished with the endoscope are emerging. New medications for sedation and analgesia are either under investigation or already are on the market. Standards for monitoring and criteria for discharge are improving.

Because of these changes, anesthesiologists have become involved in the care of many of these patients.[1] In some situations, endoscopists may not want to divide their attention between performing the procedure and maintaining the sedation. In other situations, there may be a need for more sophisticated medications that require the expertise of an anesthesiologist. Occasionally, the need for sedation is escalated, sometimes to the point of requiring general anesthesia, because of the complexity of the procedure. Last, these procedures also are becoming common in children, whose cooperation may be gained only with the administration of general anesthesia.

This article originally appeared in *Anesthesiology Clinics of North America*, Volume 27, Issue 1.
Department of Anesthesiology, University of Kentucky College of Medicine, 800 Rose Street, Lexington, KY 40536, USA
* Corresponding author.
E-mail address: dgoul0@email.uky.edu (D.T. Goulson).

Perioperative Nursing Clinics 4 (2009) 421–435
doi:10.1016/j.cpen.2009.09.008
1556-7931/09/$ – see front matter © 2009 Elsevier Inc. All rights reserved.

The provision of anesthesia or sedation for endoscopy is associated with issues that are different from care during surgical cases. Some of those areas of difference relate to the location in which the care is provided, relationships with the endoscopists, relationships with payors, varying levels of patient preparation, the use of different medications, and the management of complications in an out-of-operating-room environment. This article covers all of these areas.

VENUES

Historically, GI endoscopy was performed in a hospital setting. A recent survey of members of the American College of Gastroenterology shows this still is true most of the time. The ambulatory surgery center (ASC) now is becoming the preferred location for these procedures,[2] however, and approximately 35.8% of endoscopists consider an ASC as their primary location for performance of endoscopy.[1] There seem to be significant regional differences in where endoscopies are done. For example, office endoscopy accounted for 19.8% of procedures in the Mid-Atlantic region but only 0.4% in the Northeast in the 2004 survey.[1] Some of these differences are related to reimbursement issues,[3] and some are related to local customs and practices.

From the perspective of the anesthesiologist, the venue is important for several reasons. The most important is the capability for patient monitoring and resuscitation that is available in a particular location. Secondary considerations involve the scheduling and availability of anesthesia personnel, if requested for assistance in the sedation. Most anesthesiologists believe that an operating room provides the most flexibility for caring for medically challenging patients. Endoscopy equipment is relatively portable, compared with the equipment for other nonsurgical procedures in which anesthesiologists are involved (eg, CT scanning). This portability makes it possible for endoscopy cases to be treated in an operating room even if that location is not the endoscopist's preference.

SEDATION VERSUS GENERAL ANESTHESIA

In the survey mentioned previously, gastroenterologists in the United States reported that sedation is provided for 98% to 99% of esophagogastroduodenoscopies (EGDs) and colonoscopies.[1] It seems likely that this nearly universal use of sedation also is the practice for other procedures performed in the GI suite, such as endoscopic retrograde cholangiopancreatography (ERCP) and endoscopic ultrasonography (EUS). Most patients received sedation under the supervision of the gastroenterologist; the survey reported that anesthesia care providers (both anesthesiologists and certified registered nurse anesthetists) were responsible for providing sedation in approximately 28% of cases. Of note, the use of anesthesia personnel varies widely among geographic areas. Fewer than 10% of patients undergoing procedures in the Northeast, Midwest, and Southwest regions have an anesthesia care provider involved in their care, but 17% of patients in the South and more than one third of patients in the Mid-Atlantic area have anesthesia professionals responsible for administering their sedation. Some of these regional differences may be economically driven and are discussed later in this article. Although are no data are available to describe what patient characteristics prompt the GI physician to use anesthesia professionals, the experience of most anesthesiologists is that they are asked to care primarily for pediatric patients, patients who have a history of being difficult to sedate, and patients who have life-threatening medical conditions.

When anesthetizing patients in the GI suite, an anesthesiologist first must decide what level of sedation or anesthesia is required. Many factors play a role in this decision-making process. The patient's medical status, including whether the patient is at risk for aspiration and requires protection of the airway with an endotracheal tube, is an essential factor to consider. The complexity of the GI procedure, the patient position required to perform the procedure, and the proximity of the anesthesia care provider to the patient's airway during the procedure also must be considered when developing an anesthetic plan. Other factors that often are used in this decision-making process include a patient's history of failed sedation by non-anesthesia health care providers, substance abuse, or mental illness.

Relatively healthy patients who are undergoing simpler procedures, such as EGD or colonoscopy, often tolerate the procedure well with moderate sedation. At many institutions these patients are sedated without the involvement of anesthesia personnel. A significant number of GI facilities, however, do use anesthesia care providers for nearly all sedation procedures, and anesthesiologists can expect to provide moderate sedation to the most of their patients in such a practice setting. In most GI units, however, anesthesia professionals usually are involved only for more complex patients or procedures. These situations often require deep sedation or general anesthesia to achieve adequate patient comfort, cooperation, and optimal operating conditions for the GI physician.

One challenge for both gastroenterologists and anesthesiologists is to predict before the procedure which patients will require deep sedation or general anesthesia not because of the patient's medical condition or the complexity of the procedure but to provide sufficient patient cooperation and comfort. Data to determine patient factors that could assist in identifying patients who may be difficult to sedate do not seem to be available and could be the focus of future study. In areas outside North America, many patients undergo simple GI procedures, such as EGD, without any sedation. There are data from Europe identifying factors that predict poor patient tolerance of an unsedated EGD, and these same patient characteristics also might predict patients who will require deeper levels of sedation or general anesthesia for a successful procedure in practice settings where sedation is used for all patients. Both apprehension about the procedure, as rated by the patient, and high levels of anxiety, as measured by administering the state trait anxiety inventory before the procedure, were associated with poor patient tolerance.[4]

OTHER PRACTICAL ISSUES
Scheduling

Facility scheduling for endoscopic procedures shares many characteristics with scheduling for surgical procedures. One consideration is the availability of multiple resources, including the endoscopist, nursing personnel, endoscopy equipment, and a physical location for the procedure. Some gastroenterologists favor an open-access model of scheduling[5] in which patients are referred from other physicians and there is no preprocedure office visit. This method does present challenges in assuring that the proper procedure is indicated and that the patient is prepared adequately.

If the gastroenterology practice uses an anesthesiologist to provide sedation for only selected cases, the matter of scheduling becomes even more complicated. The availability of an anesthesiologist then must be considered as an additional resource that must be scheduled. Cases requiring the service of an anesthesiologist should be grouped together when possible to increase the likelihood of financial viability for that provider. If the volume of sedation cases is large enough, an anesthesiologist may dedicate the entire day to the endoscopy facility. Otherwise, the anesthesiologist probably will spend part of the day providing sedation for endoscopies and part of the day providing anesthesia in another location.

Preprocedure Evaluation

If the expectation is that the anesthesiologist will provide deep sedation or general anesthesia for a patient, the principles of pre-anesthetic evaluation that apply to surgical cases should apply to these endoscopic cases also. This evaluation requires a significant amount of communication between the anesthesiologist and the gastroenterologist about the patients in question. If there is a well-defined process, the patient must follow the same steps for evaluation. Depending on the patient's condition, these steps could include laboratory testing and EKG and echocardiographic evaluations. If processes for routine performance of a pre-anesthetic evaluation are not in place, the anesthesiologist must ensure that the gastroenterologist understands the expectations regarding pre-anesthetic evaluation.

The pre-anesthetic evaluation has become one of the challenges of providing anesthesia for these cases. Often the patient arrives in the facility for monitored anesthesia care or general anesthesia poorly prepared for an anesthetic. This situation results in frustration for everyone involved.

One area of particular concern is management of antiplatelet medications, especially when patients have had recent placement of a drug-eluting stent. This concern is pertinent in procedures in which there is a chance for bleeding, such as banding of esophageal varices or ERCP with sphincterotomy. As with surgical cases, the decision of whether to withhold these medications is complex and must be made in collaboration with the cardiologist, gastroenterologist, and anesthesiologist. One approach that has been advocated when patients are taking anticoagulants[6] is to perform an initial diagnostic endoscopy for visualization only while the still patient is following the usual anticoagulant regimen. Once the results of that endoscopy are known, an informed decision can be made about managing anticoagulation if a therapeutic endoscopy is needed. It is reassuring that a small case-control study of ERCP with sphincterotomy suggested that the risk of clinically significant bleeding is not increased in patients who have been taking antiplatelet medications within 10 days of the procedure.[7]

Reimbursement for Sedation and Analgesia

In the traditional model in which the gastroenterologist administers sedation, payors typically do not provide separate reimbursement for the sedation. As anesthesiologists have begun to provide this service, separate claims are being submitted for the sedation. Estimates are that charges to Medicare for anesthesia for colonoscopy increased by 86% between 2001 and 2003, to $80,000,000.[3] In response to that rapid rise, payment for anesthesia for endoscopy has been scrutinized. Most payors distinguish between high-risk and average-risk cases. In general, they have allowed charges for anesthesia in high-risk patients. Payment policies for average-risk patients are evolving, however, and there are differences among Medicare contractors. Consequently, regional differences in practice have developed that seem to be influenced by reimbursement patterns. For example, the growth in charges by anesthesiologists to Empire Medicare Services[3] in the metropolitan New York area is far steeper than the national growth rate, presumably in part because at this Medicare contractor's policies allow reimbursement.

MEDICATIONS FOR SEDATION AND ANALGESIA

The most widely used combination for sedation for GI endoscopy is a benzodiazepine, such as midazolam, and an opioid, such as meperidine or fentanyl,[8] but several other medications have been explored in the quest for ease of titration, rapid recovery, and minimization of untoward side effects.[9]

Propofol

Propofol is an agent that typically has been used for general anesthesia, but in subhypnotic doses it can produce moderate levels of sedation. Its therapeutic window is very narrow, making it easy to move from the level of moderate sedation into deep sedation or general anesthesia. Therefore the Food and Drug Administration (FDA) product label currently states that propofol "should only be administered by persons trained in the administration of general anesthesia," which also would give them the ability to rescue a patient from unintended levels of deep sedation.[10] This practice also is consistent with the Joint Commission for the Accreditation of Health Care Organization's current approach to sedation. Their standards state that practitioners providing sedation should be able to rescue patients who slip into a deeper-than-desired level of sedation.[11] Specifically, persons providing moderate sedation should be qualified to rescue patients from deep sedation and be competent to manage a compromised airway and provide adequate oxygenation and ventilation.

The drive to use propofol as an adjunct to endoscopy goes hand-in-hand with the increased demand for these procedures. Because the practice of endoscopists has become busier, there are increased needs for efficiency.[9] In the past, prolonged recovery and relatively long discharge times resulted in a loss of efficiency. Because propofol has a fast onset and allows rapid recovery, gastroenterologists have become interested in using it for their procedures. The restrictions mentioned previously, however, suggest that an anesthesiologist should be involved in the sedation.

These governmental restrictions are not as clear-cut in other countries. Quoting a worldwide experience with gastroenterologist-directed administration of propofol for procedural sedation in 200,000 patient encounters with no mortalities, several gastroenterology-related professional societies have questioned the medical necessity of restricting its use to anesthesiologists.[8] In 2005, the American College of Gastroenterology petitioned the United States FDA to remove the section of the warning label pertaining to administration by individuals trained in general anesthesia.[12]

In response to the current political and regulatory environment and in combination with escalating costs associated with administering propofol by an anesthesiologist in the United States, several alternative models of administration have emerged.[13] One alternative is nurse-administered propofol sedation. In this model, propofol is administered by registered nurses under a strict protocol and under the supervision of the endoscopist.[14] There are several studies of this model in the literature, covering more than 200,000 administrations. Questions still remain about the true incidences of airway complications[13] and need for airway interventions. Debate also continues about whether this model obviates the need for the endoscopist to have skills in deep sedation and airway rescue.

Another alternative model for propofol administration is patient-controlled sedation. The theoretic advantage of patient-controlled sedation is that it allows the patient to match his or her sedation needs to the discomfort of the procedure while avoiding the effects of oversedation.[13] This model is discussed further later in this article.

Fospropofol

Fospropofol is a water-soluble prodrug of propofol that currently is being evaluated as a sedative agent for diagnostic and therapeutic procedures.[15] It is hydrolyzed rapidly to release propofol. Following intravenous (IV) administration, the plasma concentration profile of fospropofol-derived propofol is characterized by a smooth and predictable rise and decline instead of the rapid spike observed following administration of the lipid-emulsion formulation of propofol. The elimination kinetics of propofol is similar, whether it was derived from fospropofol or not.

One dose-ranging study appears in the literature. Cohen[15] studied 127 patients receiving either midazolam or one of four different doses of fospropofol for sedation for elective colonoscopy. The investigators examined rates of sedation success, time to sedation, requirements for alternative sedative medication, requirements for assisted ventilation, supplemental doses of sedative, time to discharge, and satisfaction of the physician with the sedation. Only one patient required any kind of airway intervention, and that was verbal stimulation to address hypoxemia. The investigators concluded that the 6.5-mg/kg dose provided the ideal balance of efficacy and safety.

The medication is currently under phase III trials and has not yet been approved for use in the United States. Interestingly, the American Society of Anesthesiologists has submitted formal comments to the FDA requesting that the fospropofol label contain restrictions similar to those for propofol,[16] because they believe that this drug also will be able to produce a state of general anesthesia in patients.

Dexmedetomidine

Dexmedetomidine is another relatively new agent that has been considered for sedation for endoscopy. It is a highly selective α_2-adrenoreceptor agonist with sedative and analgesic effects[17] that was approved in 1999 by the FDA for sedation in patients in ICUs.[18] One significant reported advantage is that patients can be sedated but are able to be roused to full consciousness easily.[19]

Only a handful of studies have examined this agent specifically in the setting of endoscopy. Demiraran and colleagues[20] compared dexmedetomidine and midazolam as the sedative agent for EGD. No opioids were given in this small study of 50 patients that was performed in Turkey. The investigators concluded that dexmedetomidine and midazolam have similar efficacy and safety profiles.

Another study from Poland examined dexmedetomidine in comparison with meperidine or fentanyl as a single agent for sedation for colonoscopy. The investigators found that patients in the dexmedetomidine group required significant supplemental fentanyl and had a high risk of bradycardia and hypotension. They concluded was that dexmedetomidine is not a suitable agent for sedation.[21]

Ketamine

Ketamine has been examined both as a sole agent and in combination with other medications in adults and children. Most references in the literature relate to its use in children. Gilger and colleagues[22] retrospectively examined 402 procedures in which various combinations of midazolam, meperidine, and ketamine were used. They found that the midazolam/ketamine combination had the lowest rate of complications and a rate of adequate sedation equivalent to that of the other combinations. Intramuscular ketamine also has been studied as a sole agent for sedation in pediatric endoscopy but was found to have a high failure rate in a small study.[23] Kirberg and colleagues[24] have described their experience with ketamine in both pediatric endoscopy and adult endoscopy and have found it to be an effective agent. In advanced endoscopic procedures in adults, such as ERCP and EUS, ketamine is a useful adjunct to more traditional sedation agents and helps produce acceptable procedural conditions.[25]

Benzodiazepines

Benzodiazepines have long been an integral part of the sedation regimen for GI endoscopy. The early preparations of IV benzodiazepines were lipid soluble, creating issues with administration. During that time, diazepam was the medication in this class most frequently used for endoscopy. Once water-soluble midazolam became available in the late 1980s, it quickly gained favor.[26] Today, midazolam is strongly favored over diazepam.[1]

Opioids

The second part of the conventional sedation combination is an opioid. Twenty years ago, meperidine was a mainstay.[26] Today, meperidine and fentanyl are used about equally.[1] Some practitioners also have begun to use other fast-acting opioids such as remifentanil,[27] although usually not as a single agent.

SEDATION/ANESTHESIA FOR SPECIFIC PROCEDURES

GI endoscopic procedures vary significantly in their complexity and the degree of patient stimulation and pain that occur. Therefore, the optimal sedation or anesthetic techniques for various procedures for various procedures differ.

Esophagogastroduodenoscopy

Adequate sedation for EGD can be achieved in most patients with a combination of an IV benzodiazepine and opioid, but most anesthesiologists use IV propofol for EGD sedations. When surveyed, gastroenterologists have reported greater satisfaction with propofol than with the conventional sedation technique of benzodiazepine and an opioid. In fact, the median satisfaction score for propofol was 10 on a 10-point scale in which 10 was defined as best.[1] Moderate and deep sedation as well as general anesthesia can be achieved with propofol. Patients who have a history of substance abuse or of being difficult to sedate usually require deep sedation or general anesthesia for an EGD procedure. Even when moderate sedation is the intended goal for the procedure, however, deep sedation often is achieved. In one study, 60% of patients undergoing EGD reached a level of deep sedation despite a preprocedure plan for moderate sedation.[28]

Another factor to consider when choosing between sedation and general anesthesia for EGD is whether endotracheal intubation is needed. The indication for performing EGD, such as persistent vomiting or severe gastroesophageal reflux disease, may dictate protection of the airway with an endotracheal tube. In other patients, such as those who are obese or who have obstructive sleep apnea, significant airway obstruction during deep sedation may necessitate endotracheal intubation. Patients who do undergo endotracheal intubation usually require a level of general anesthesia to tolerate adequately both the endoscopic procedure and the presence of the endotracheal tube.

A unique anesthetic technique for EGD that has been reported is general anesthesia via a ProSeal laryngeal mask airway (LMA).[29] The drain tube of this specialized LMA can serve as a conduit to guide the gastroscope into the stomach, thus possibly improving the ease of the endoscopic procedure for the gastroenterologist. In the recent study that described this technique, the anesthesia and endoscopy times were significantly shorter in the group of patients randomly assigned to the use of the ProSeal LMA than in patients who received the same anesthetic drugs but whose airways were managed with chin lift/jaw thrust as needed and oxygen via nasal cannula. In addition, the mean oxygen saturation was higher and fewer episodes of arterial oxyhemoglobin saturation (SpO_2) less than 90% occurred in the ProSeal group than in the nasal cannula group.

An adjunct to sedation for EGD that often is overlooked but should be considered by anesthesiologists is topical pharyngeal anesthesia. Although some studies have reported no added benefit from topical anesthesia in sedated patients,[30] other individual studies[31] as well as a meta-analysis[32] have reported that ease of endoscopy is improved in patients who receive topical pharyngeal anesthesia in addition to sedation. In the United States, commercially available local anesthetic sprays, including Cetacaine and Hurricane sprays, are used most commonly to provide pharyngeal anesthesia. These sprays contain benzocaine, which has been associated with the development of methemoglobinemia.[33] Another option for topical anesthesia that could avoid the risk of methemoglobinemia is use of a lidocaine lollipop. Investigators at an institution in Lebanon found this technique very effective. In fact, only one third of patients who received the lollipop required IV sedation for EGD, whereas nearly 100% of the patients who did not receive topical anesthesia required sedation.[34]

Colonoscopy

Like EGD, adequate sedation for colonoscopy can be achieved with a combination of benzodiazepine and an opioid in most patients. One study found that when moderate sedation was planned, deep sedation was less likely to be achieved during colonoscopy than during EGD, ERCP, or EUS.[28] This difference may be explained by the apparently less stimulating nature of colonoscopy compared with the other procedures. When anesthesia professionals provide sedation for colonoscopy, however, they usually use propofol and often plan to attain a level of deep sedation or general anesthesia. In fact, it seems likely that even when gastroenterologists are responsible for the sedation during colonoscopy, they and their patients actually prefer to achieve at least deep sedation rather than moderate sedation. In a study of nurse-administered propofol sedation that was performed under the supervision of the GI physician, the mean bispectral index score was 59, indicating a state of general anesthesia.[35]

Several sedation or anesthesia techniques for colonoscopy have been studied. Remifentanil is a very short-acting opioid that may offer advantages for patients undergoing outpatient colonoscopy. Moerman and colleagues[36] compared IV remifentanil versus IV propofol. They found that measures of early recovery, such as spontaneous eye opening and following commands, occurred sooner in the patients who received remifentanil. Recovery of cognitive function also was faster with remifentanil than with propofol. Respiratory depression occurred more frequently in the remifentanil group, however, and patient satisfaction was lower in this group than in the propofol group. In another study that compared remifentanil and propofol, postprocedure nausea and vomiting was a significant problem with remifentanil sedation.[37] General anesthesia using an inhalational technique of sevoflurane/nitrous oxide has been compared with total IV anesthesia (TIVA) using propofol/fentanyl/midazolam for colonoscopy. Patients who received the inhalational anesthetic were less sedated 20 minutes after the procedure than patients who received TIVA. A greater degree of psychomotor impairment that lasted longer also was reported in the TIVA group.[38]

The use of propofol alone to achieve deep sedation has been compared with lower doses of propofol in combination with fentanyl and/or midazolam titrated to moderate sedation. Patients who received the combination therapy were discharged more quickly than patients who received only propofol with no differences found between the groups in satisfaction scores, vital signs, or oxygen saturation.[39]

Patient-controlled sedation with propofol is a new technique that seems to be effective for sedation during colonoscopy. A prospective, randomized study in France compared patient-controlled sedation with anesthesiologist-administered propofol. Patients in the patient-controlled group self-administered 20-mg boluses of propofol as needed with a lock-out time of 1 minute. Patients in the anesthesiologist-controlled group received a continuous infusion of propofol that was titrated to effect. Success of the colonoscopy, which was defined by reaching the cecum, and technical ease of the procedure as rated by the gastroenterologist did not differ between the groups. In addition, patient satisfaction was similar between the groups. Several advantages were reported for patient-controlled propofol administration compared with administration by an anesthesiologist. Depth of sedation was less in the patient-controlled group, and fewer episodes of SpO_2 less than 94% were reported. Time to discharge also was shorter with patient-controlled sedation. The most striking difference reported was the mean total dose of propofol administered: 60 mg in the patient-controlled group versus 248 mg in the physician-administered group.[40] It is quite probable that patient-controlled sedation may become a preferred method of sedation for colonoscopy in the future.

Endoscopic Retrograde Cholangiopancreatography

Patients undergoing ERCP often are more severely ill than patients undergoing EGD or colonoscopy. Common presenting diagnoses include pancreatitis, pancreatic cancer, and cholangitis. The serious medical conditions of these patients may account in part for the high risk of cardiopulmonary complications associated with ERCP. In one study of patients cared for by anesthesia care providers, approximately 25% of patients age 65 years or older developed new electrocardiographic changes during or after ERCP, and 11% of patients in that age group had elevated cardiac troponin levels after the procedure.[41] Relatively complex therapeutic procedures that are of longer duration than EGD or colonoscopy, such as biliary sphincterotomy, removal of bile duct stones, and placement of biliary stents, frequently are undertaken during the ERCP. Patient immobility is an important factor in the successful completion of these technically challenging procedures. Most endoscopists perform ERCP in the prone position. Finally, some of these patients require chronic opioid therapy because of their underlying biliary disease. Therefore, management of patients presenting for ERCP often is more challenging for the anesthesiologist than providing anesthesia for EGD or colonoscopy.

Despite these challenges, some anesthesiologists successfully provide moderate or deep sedation for ERCP. Propofol usually is the preferred sedative drug. One study compared sedation with midazolam or propofol. The procedure was completed successfully more often in patients receiving propofol (97.5%, vs 80% for midazolam), and recovery time was significantly shorter.[42] Anesthesiologists also have provided successful sedation for ERCP by using a target-controlled infusion of propofol and titrating to a target concentration of 2 to 5 μg/mL.[43]

Several of these issues encountered with ERCP have led many anesthesiologists to prefer general anesthesia for this procedure. There are data that support this clinical approach. In one retrospective study of more than 1000 patients, the ERCP failure rate with moderate sedation was double that with general anesthesia (14% vs 7%), with most failures resulting from inadequate sedation.[44] It also has been reported that complication rates associated with therapeutic interventions during ERCP may be significantly lower when general anesthesia is used, perhaps because the absence of patient movement makes the procedure technically less difficult.[45]

When general anesthesia is administered for ERCP, the airway often is protected by endotracheal intubation because of the prone position required during the procedure and because of the presence of risk factors for aspiration in some patients. Investigators, however, have used the LMA successfully for ERCP performed under general anesthesia, in some cases even placing the LMA while the patient was in the prone position. They reported that the endoscope was advanced without difficulty, and time to removal of the airway device was shorter than in patients who underwent endotracheal intubation.[46]

Endoscopic Ultrasonography

Like ERCP, EUS is a more complex procedure than EGD or colonoscopy. It is used for diagnosing and staging GI and pancreatic tumors. Needle-aspiration biopsies often are performed that require examination by a pathologist to determine the adequacy of the sample before the procedure can be completed. Therefore, EUS procedures may be relatively long in duration. In addition, the specialized ultrasound-containing endoscope is significantly larger than a standard endoscope, and insertion causes more patient discomfort than experienced during EGD. As a result, adequate sedation for the procedure is more likely to require deep sedation or general anesthesia.

Some patients satisfactorily tolerate an EUS procedure with a combination of benzodiazepine and an opioid. Titration to an adequate level of sedation while avoiding airway obstruction and hypoxemia may be more problematic during EUS than during EGD or colonoscopy, however. As a result, alternative sedation techniques have been investigated. In one study, preprocedure sedation with moderate doses of benzodiazepine and an opioid were supplemented as needed during the EUS with either ketamine or additional doses of the benzodiazepine and opioid. Improved sedation (as measured by patient comfort and degree of sedation-related technical difficulty) and faster recovery were achieved with ketamine. In addition, approximately one third of patients who were assigned randomly to the benzodiazepine/opioid arm of the study had to cross over to ketamine to achieve an adequate level of sedation to complete the EUS successfully.[25]

Propofol, of course, is another preferred anesthetic drug for EUS. A propofol infusion controlled manually by the anesthesiologist is used most commonly, but other techniques, including a target-controlled propofol infusion, have been used successfully for sedation during EUS. Because preprocedure anxiolysis is beneficial in some patients, one group of investigators studied the effect of administering a dose of midazolam before initiating the target-controlled infusion. Administration of midazolam did not reduce significantly the amount of propofol required during the EUS, but it also did not delay the time to discharge readiness.[47] Patient-controlled sedation with propofol and fentanyl, using 4.25-mg boluses of propofol and 3.75-μg boluses of fentanyl without a lock-out time, also has provided sedation successfully during EUS.[48]

Pediatric Procedures

Most pediatric patients require deep sedation or general anesthesia to tolerate GI endoscopic procedures. Therefore, anesthesiologists are more likely to participate in pediatric procedures than in adult procedures. At many institutions, anesthesia care providers administer the sedation or anesthesia for all or most pediatric endoscopies. Many of the anesthetic principles and drugs used in caring for adult GI patients are pertinent in the pediatric population, but there are additional challenges. Typically, pediatric patients require larger per-weight doses of the sedative medications than adults. One group of investigators determined the median effective concentration of propofol required for EGD in children. It was significantly higher (3.55 µg/mL) than the usual concentration required in adults undergoing this procedure.[49]

Other challenges encountered when caring for children in the GI suite that are unique to the pediatric population are distress caused by the insertion of an IV catheter and by separation from parents. When young children are anesthetized in the operating room, IV catheters usually are placed after mask induction with a volatile anesthetic agent. At many GI facilities, it is not practical to have an anesthesia machine available, and IV drugs are used to provide both sedation and general anesthesia. Insertion of the IV catheter often is the most difficult part of the sedation procedure for everyone involved (patient, parents, and practitioner). Techniques that can facilitate IV placement as well as separation from the parents are invaluable. In one study, preprocedure administration of oral midazolam was more effective in improving both concerns than the use of IV propofol only. The researchers also found that administration of oral midazolam significantly decreased the dose of propofol required during endoscopy. Recovery time was significantly longer in patients who received midazolam, but longer recovery time seems a small price to pay to make the procedure less traumatic for both child and parents, especially because the mean recovery time still was only 26 minutes.[50]

MANAGING COMPLICATIONS

One prospective cohort study has reported on cardiopulmonary complications that occurred during nearly 12,000 colonoscopies or EGDs in which patients received monitored anesthesia care with propofol. The overall rate of complications was 0.86% for colonoscopy and 1.01% for EGD. The rate of serious adverse events was much lower, however: 13 of 8129 colonoscopies and 6 of 3762 EGDs. Of interest, the rate of complications was lower for both procedures when an anesthesia practitioner, rather than a gastroenterologist, provided sedation.[51] There are few other data available about sedation or anesthesia-related complications associated with GI endoscopy when sedation was provided by an anesthesiologist.

Despite the limited data, anesthesiologists should anticipate that anesthetic complications will occur occasionally. The principles for management of these complications do not differ from management in the operating room, but anesthesia practitioners also must realize that the resources available for handling these problems in the operating room suite may not be as readily accessible in the endoscopy suite. Support personnel in the operating room may be comfortable assisting anesthesiologists during acute cardiopulmonary events, but nursing staff in the GI suite have more limited exposure to such events and may not be able to provide the same level of assistance. Necessary equipment, such as that needed for advanced airway techniques, may not be available immediately. Before providing anesthesia services in the endoscopy unit, the anesthesiologist should anticipate, based on the patient's medical condition, what equipment might be needed and have it present in the GI suite. The anesthesiologist also should have a plan for obtaining additional assistance in the event of a serious adverse event. Many of these endoscopy procedures can be performed in an operating room. In certain high-risk patients, it is appropriate to request that the anesthetizing location be moved to the operating room where serious anesthesia-related complications can be managed more efficiently and effectively.

POSTANESTHESIA RECOVERY

At facilities where most endoscopy procedures are performed with gastroenterologist-administered moderate sedation, the anesthesiologist must understand fully the capabilities of the nursing staff responsible for monitoring patients during the recovery period. These units sometimes are equipped only to provide nursing care at the level necessary for monitoring patients who have received moderate sedation. It is essential that patients who have received deep sedation or general anesthesia for their endoscopy procedures receive the same level of nursing care they would in the postanesthesia care unit (PACU) of the institution's surgical suite. In fact, regulatory organizations such as the Joint Commission for Accreditation of Health Care Organizations require that equivalent postanesthesia care be delivered in all locations within the health care facility. Information such as the type of training the recovery nurses in the endoscopy suite have received (eg, is the training equivalent to that required of nurses who work in the surgical postanesthesia care unit?) and whether the same patient/nurse staffing ratio used in the surgical PACU can be achieved in the GI suite must be determined when deciding on the appropriate location for recovery of these patients. If adequate nursing care is available, it is preferable for the postanesthesia recovery to occur in the endoscopy suite to avoid transportation of the patient to another location in the immediate postprocedure period. If the anesthesia care provider does not feel comfortable with the level of care available in the GI suite, however, arrangements to transfer the patient to the surgical suite's PACU should be made. Even when satisfactory recovery room care is available in the endoscopy suite, it may be advisable to monitor patients who are at especially high risk for developing anesthesia-related complications in a unit such as the surgical suite's PACU, where these complications are encountered and managed on a frequent basis.

Discharge criteria should be the same as those used for patients who receive anesthesia or sedation in the operating room. Recovery nurses need to understand fully the criteria and know how to contact anesthesia personnel for assistance during the recovery period. Postanesthesia management of patients who have obstructive sleep apnea may be especially challenging. Based on the guidelines published by the American Society of Anesthesiologists,[52] it should be expected that prolonged recovery times may be required for these patients. If logistical or staffing issues do not allow extended monitoring of these patients, arrangements for postanesthesia recovery in another location will be necessary.

REFERENCES

1. Cohen LB, Wecsler JS, Gaetano JN, et al. Endoscopic sedation in the United States: results from a nationwide survey. Am J Gastroenterol 2006;101:967–74.
2. Frakes JT. Outpatient endoscopy. The case for the ambulatory surgery center. Gastrointest Endosc Clin N Am 2002;12:215–27.
3. Aisenberg J, Brill JV, Ladabaum U, et al. Sedation for gastrointestinal endoscopy: new practices, new economics. Am J Gastroenterol 2005;100:996–1000.
4. Campo R, Brullet E, Montserrat A, et al. Identification of factors that influence tolerance of upper gastrointestinal endoscopy. Eur J Gastroenterol Hepatol 1999;11:201–4.
5. Pike IM. Open-access endoscopy. Gastrointest Endosc Clin N Am 2006;16: 709–17.

6. Mathew A, Riley TR 3rd, Young M, et al. Cost-saving approach to patients on long-term anticoagulation who need endoscopy: a decision analysis. Am J Gastroenterol 2003;98:1766–76.

7. Hussain N, Alsulaiman R, Burtin P, et al. The safety of endoscopic sphincterotomy in patients receiving antiplatelet agents—a case-control study. Aliment Pharmacol Ther 2007;25:579–84.

8. Cohen LB, Delegge MH, Aisenberg J, et al. AGA Institute review of endoscopic sedation. Gastroenterology 2007;133:675–701.

9. Vargo JJ, Bramley T, Meyer K, et al. Practice efficiency and economics: the case for rapid recovery sedation agents for colonoscopy in a screening population. J Clin Gastroenterol 2007;41:591–8.

10. Food and Drug Administration. Propofol draft final printed label. Available at: http://www.fda.gov/cder/foi/anda/2000/75392_Propofol_Prntlbl.pdf. Accessed June 1, 2008.

11. Comprehensive accreditation manual for hospitals. Oakbrook Terrace (IL): Joint Commission on Accreditation of Healthcare Organizations; 2008.

12. Aisenberg J, Cohen LB, Piorkowski JD. Propofol use under the direction of trained gastroenterologists: an analysis of the medicolegal implications. CME. Am J Gastroenterol 2007;102:707–13.

13. Trummel J. Sedation for gastrointestinal endoscopy: the changing landscape. Curr Opin Anaesthesiol 2007;20:359–64.

14. Rex DK, Overley CA, Walker J. Registered nurse-administered propofol sedation for upper endoscopy and colonoscopy: why? when? how? Rev Gastroenterol Disord 2003;3:70–80.

15. Cohen LB. Clinical trial: a dose-response study of fospropofol disodium for moderate sedation during colonoscopy. Aliment Pharmacol Ther 2008;27:597–608.

16. American Society of Anesthesiologists. ASA comments at FDA hearing on fospropofol. Available at: http://www.asahq.org/news/asanews050808.htm. Accessed June 1, 2008.

17. Aantaa R, Scheinin M. Alpha 2-adrenergic agents in anaesthesia. Acta Anaesthesiol Scand 1993;37:433–48.

18. Venn RM, Grounds RM. Comparison between dexmedetomidine and propofol for sedation in the intensive care unit: patient and clinician perceptions. Br J Anaesth 2001;87:684–90.

19. Shelly MP. Dexmedetomidine: a real innovation or more of the same? Br J Anaesth 2001;87:677–8.

20. Demiraran Y, Korkut E, Tamer A, et al. The comparison of dexmedetomidine and midazolam used for sedation of patients during upper endoscopy: a prospective, randomized study. Can J Gastroenterol 2007;21:25–9.

21. Jalowiecki P, Rudner R, Gonciarz M, et al. Sole use of dexmedetomidine has limited utility for conscious sedation during outpatient colonoscopy. Anesthesiology 2005;103:269–73.

22. Gilger MA, Spearman RS, Dietrich CL, et al. Safety and effectiveness of ketamine as a sedative agent for pediatric GI endoscopy. Gastrointest Endosc 2004;59:659–63.

23. Law AK, Ng DK, Chan KK. Use of intramuscular ketamine for endoscopy sedation in children. Pediatr Int 2003;45:180–5.

24. Kirberg A, Sagredo R, Montalva G, et al. Ketamine for pediatric endoscopic procedures and as a sedation complement for adult patients. Gastrointest Endosc 2005;61:501–2.

25. Varadarajulu S, Eloubeidi MA, Tamhane A, et al. Prospective randomized trial evaluating ketamine for advanced endoscopic procedures in difficult to sedate patients. Aliment Pharmacol Ther 2007;25:987–97.
26. Keeffe EB, O'Connor KW. 1989 A/S/G/E survey of endoscopic sedation and monitoring practices. Gastrointest Endosc 1990;36:S13.
27. Litman RS. Conscious sedation with remifentanil during painful medical procedures. J Pain Symptom Manage 2000;19:468–71.
28. Patel S, Vargo JJ, Khandwala F, et al. Deep sedation occurs frequently during elective endoscopy with meperidine and midazolam. Am J Gastroenterol 2005; 100:2689–95.
29. Lopez-Gil M, Brimacombe J, Diaz-Reganon G. Anesthesia for pediatric gastroscopy: a study comparing the proseal laryngeal mask airway with nasal cannulae. Paediatr Anaesth 2006;16:1032–5.
30. Davis DE, Jones MP, Kubik CM. Topical pharyngeal anesthesia does not improve upper gastrointestinal endoscopy in conscious sedated patients. Am J Gastroenterol 1999;94:1853–6.
31. Ristikankare M, Hartikainen J, Heikkinen M, et al. Is routine sedation or topical pharyngeal anesthesia beneficial during upper endoscopy? Gastrointest Endosc 2004;60:686–94.
32. Evans LT, Saberi S, Kim HM, et al. Pharyngeal anesthesia during sedated EGDs: is "the spray" beneficial? A meta-analysis and systematic review. Gastrointest Endosc 2006;63:761–6.
33. Byrne MF, Mitchell RM, Gerke H, et al. The need for caution with topical anesthesia during endoscopic procedures, as liberal use may result in methemoglobinemia. J Clin Gastroenterol 2004;38:225–9.
34. Ayoub C, Skoury A, Abdul-Baki H, et al. Lidocaine lollipop as single-agent anesthesia in upper GI endoscopy. Gastrointest Endosc 2007;66:786–93.
35. Chen SC, Rex DK. An initial investigation of bispectral monitoring as an adjunct to nurse-administered propofol sedation for colonoscopy. Am J Gastroenterol 2004; 99:1081–6.
36. Moerman AT, Foubert LA, Herregods LL, et al. Propofol versus remifentanil for monitored anaesthesia care during colonoscopy. Eur J Anaesthesiol 2003;20:461–6.
37. Akcaboy ZN, Akcaboy EY, Albayrak D, et al. Can remifentanil be a better choice than propofol for colonoscopy during monitored anesthesia care? Acta Anaesthesiol Scand 2006;50:736–41.
38. Theodorou T, Hales P, Gillespie P, et al. Total intravenous versus inhalational anaesthesia for colonoscopy: a prospective study of clinical recovery and psychomotor function. Anaesth Intensive Care 2001;29:124–36.
39. VanNatta ME, Rex DK. Propofol alone titrated to deep sedation versus propofol in combination with opioids and/or benzodiazepines and titrated to moderate sedation for colonoscopy. Am J Gastroenterol 2006;101:2209–17.
40. Crepeau T, Poincloux L, Bonny C, et al. Significance of patient-controlled sedation during colonoscopy. Results from a prospective randomized controlled study. Gastroenterol Clin Biol 2005;29:1090–6.
41. Fisher L, Fisher A, Thomson A. Cardiopulmonary complications of ERCP in older patients. Gastrointest Endosc 2006;63:948–55.
42. Jung M, Hofmann C, Kiesslich R, et al. Improved sedation in diagnostic and therapeutic ERCP: propofol is an alternative to midazolam. Endoscopy 2000;32:233–8.
43. Fanti L, Agostoni M, Casati A, et al. Target-controlled propofol infusion during monitored anesthesia in patients undergoing ERCP. Gastrointest Endosc 2004; 60:361–6.

44. Raymondos K, Panning B, Bachem I, et al. Evaluation of endoscopic retrograde cholangiopancreatography under conscious sedation and general anesthesia. Endoscopy 2002;34:721–6.
45. Martindale SJ. Anaesthetic considerations during endoscopic retrograde cholangiopancreatography. Anaesth Intensive Care 2006;34:475–80.
46. Osborn IP, Cohen J, Soper RJ, et al. Laryngeal mask airway—a novel method of airway protection during ERCP: comparison with endotracheal intubation. Gastrointest Endosc 2002;56:122–8.
47. Fanti L, Agostoni M, Arcidiacono PG, et al. Target-controlled infusion during monitored anesthesia care in patients undergoing EUS: propofol alone versus midazolam plus propofol. A prospective double-blind randomised controlled trial. Dig Liver Dis 2007;39:81–6.
48. Agostoni M, Fanti L, Arcidiacono PG, et al. Midazolam and pethidine versus propofol and fentanyl patient controlled sedation/analgesia for upper gastrointestinal tract ultrasound endoscopy: a prospective randomized controlled trial. Dig Liver Dis 2007;39:1024–9.
49. Hammer GB, Litalien C, Wellis V, et al. Determination of the median effective concentration (EC50) of propofol during oesophagogastroduodenoscopy in children. Paediatr Anaesth 2001;11:549–53.
50. Paspatis GA, Charoniti I, Manolaraki M, et al. Synergistic sedation with oral midazolam as a premedication and intravenous propofol versus intravenous propofol alone in upper gastrointestinal endoscopies in children: a prospective, randomized study. J Pediatr Gastroenterol Nutr 2006;43:195–9.
51. Vargo JJ, Holub JL, Faigel DO, et al. Risk factors for cardiopulmonary events during propofol-mediated upper endoscopy and colonoscopy. Aliment Pharmacol Ther 2006;24:955–63.
52. Gross JB, Bachenberg KL, Benumof JL, et al. Practice guidelines for the perioperative management of patients with obstructive sleep apnea: a report by the American society of anesthesiologists task force on perioperative management of patients with obstructive sleep apnea. Anesthesiology 2006;104:1081–93.

Anesthesiology and Gastroenterology

Willem J.S. de Villiers, MD, PhD, MHCM

KEYWORDS

- Gastroenterologist-directed propofol • NOTES • Halo system
- Endoscopic mucosal resection • Deep balloon enteroscopy
- Chromoendoscopy

Sedation and analgesia are considered by many gastroenterologists to be integral components of the endoscopic examination. For example, more than 98% of endoscopists in the United States routinely administer sedation during upper and lower endoscopies.[1] Sedation is intended primarily to reduce a patient's anxiety and discomfort, consequently improving their tolerability and satisfaction for the procedure. Endoscopic sedation also minimizes a patient's risk of physical injury during an examination and provides the endoscopist with an ideal environment for a thorough examination. Despite the benefits of sedation, its use remains problematic. Sedation delays patient recovery and discharge, adds to the overall cost of an endoscopic procedure, and increases the risk of cardiopulmonary complications. Notwithstanding these considerations, the use of sedation during endoscopy continues to increase throughout the world.[1,2]

The high costs of providing anesthesia by specialists and the relative lack of specialist personnel in many countries have led to the wider introduction of sedation delivered by nonanesthesiologists. Such sedation should be targeted for moderate levels of sedation; however, personnel should be able to avoid — and rescue patients from — deeper sedation levels. Several conditions have to be fulfilled to provide proper and safe nonanesthesiologist sedation for endoscopy, especially when propofol is to be used. These conditions include formal training, supervision by anesthesiology staff, and the definition of standard operating procedures on the national as well as local levels.

The goal of this review is (1) to provide a gastroenterology perspective on the use of propofol in gastroenterology endoscopic practice, and (2) to describe newer GI endoscopy procedures that gastroenterologists perform that might involve anesthesiologists. Mutual understanding and respect are fundamental requirements for the

This article originally appeared in *Anesthesiology Clinics of North America*, Volume 27, Issue 1.
Division of Digestive Diseases and Nutrition, Department of Internal Medicine, University of Kentucky Medical Center, University of Kentucky College of Medicine, 800 Rose Street, Room MN649, Lexington, KY 40536, USA
E-mail address: willem.devilliers@uky.edu

Perioperative Nursing Clinics 4 (2009) 437–450
doi:10.1016/j.cpen.2009.09.009

integration of gastrointestinal endoscopy and anesthesia services to optimize patient outcomes.

PROPOFOL USE IN GI ENDOSCOPY

The acceptance of colonoscopy as the gold standard modality to screen for colorectal polyps and cancer has dramatically increased the number of these procedures performed annually. There has also been an increasing emphasis on factors that could improve patient acceptance of the procedure and patient satisfaction as well as efficiency and throughput in endoscopy centers. Propofol initially was developed and approved in 1989 as a hypnotic agent for induction and maintenance of anesthesia. Accordingly, its US Food and Drug Administration (FDA) product label states "[propofol] should be administered only by persons trained in the administration of general anesthesia."[3] Since approval in the late 1980s, its clinical applications have expanded to include monitored anesthesia care and procedural sedation. Compared with conventional endoscopic sedation, it is generally accepted that propofol offers faster and more complete patient recovery, greater endoscopist and patient satisfaction, and better success with the hard-to-sedate patient.

Worldwide, the experience with gastroenterologist-directed administration of propofol now exceeds 200,000 patient experiences with no mortalities.[4–7] This, combined with improvements in our understanding of its dosing and titration for moderate sedation, have prompted several professional medical societies to question the medical necessity of restricting its use to anesthesiology professionals. The American Gastroenterological Association, the American College of Gastroenterology, and the American Society for Gastrointestinal Endoscopy all support gastroenterologist-directed administration of propofol by gastroenterologists. In a joint statement, the three societies declared that "with adequate training, physician-supervised nurse administration of propofol can be done safely and effectively."[3] However, the American Society for Anesthesiology countered that the use of propofol should be restricted to those experienced in the skills (such as endotracheal intubation) that are required during general anesthesia.[8] Much of this debate, during a time of increasing health care costs and decreasing physician reimbursements, seems to reflect economic rather than clinical concerns.[9]

Two models have emerged for the administration of propofol by endoscopists: nurse-administered propofol sedation (NAPS) and combination propofol sedation (also referred to as gastroenterologist-directed sedation). Both techniques emphasize several key principles: (1) the use of an established protocol for drug administration, (2) a sedation team with appropriate education and training, and (3) continuous patient assessment of clinical and physiologic parameters throughout the procedure.

The practice of NAPS involves a trained registered nurse whose sole responsibilities are patient monitoring and the administration of propofol. Recommendations for the initial bolus of propofol range from 10 to 60 mg, and additional boluses of 10 to 20 mg are administered with a minimum of 20 to 30 seconds between doses. Propofol dosing and the depth of sedation are individualized to the needs of each patient. Because propofol possesses no analgesic effect, many patients receiving NAPS will require deep sedation. Heart rate, blood pressure, and pulse oximetry are monitored routinely during NAPS. In most protocols, supplemental oxygen is administered to all patients.

Rex and colleageus[7] published a retrospective review of more than 36,000 endoscopies performed with NAPS at three centers, two within the United States and one in

Switzerland. The targeted depth of sedation was not specified, and the mean doses of propofol at each center were 107, 158, and 245 mg, and 144, 209, and 287 mg, during esophagogastroduodenoscopy and colonoscopy, respectively. The rate of clinically important events, defined as an episode of apnea or other airway compromise requiring assisted ventilation (bag-mask), ranged from approximately 1 per 500 to 1 per 1000. In this large case series, endotracheal intubation was not required and no patient suffered permanent injury or death.

Tohda and colleagues[10] recently reported the results of 27,500 endoscopies performed with NAPS during a 6-year period. These investigators targeted moderate rather than deep sedation. Supplemental oxygen was not provided routinely. The mean doses of propofol during esophagogastroduodenoscopy and colonoscopy were 72 and 94 mg, respectively. Notably, there were no serious cardiopulmonary events in this series, and no patient required mask ventilation, endotracheal intubation, or any form of resuscitation.

GASTROENTEROLOGIST-DIRECTED PROPOFOL SEDATION

In combination propofol sedation, also known as gastroenterologist-directed propofol sedation, the dosing responsibility is shared between the physician and nurse, and propofol is combined with very small doses of a benzodiazepine and opioid narcotic.[11] It is thus possible to maximize the desirable therapeutic actions of each agent while minimizing the likelihood of a dose-related adverse reaction. When propofol is combined with small doses of an opioid analgesic and a benzodiazepine, analgesia and amnesia can be achieved with subhypnotic doses of propofol, eliminating the need for deep sedation. Furthermore, more precise dose titration is possible with smaller bolus doses of propofol (5–15 mg), and the potential for pharmacologic reversibility is retained using naloxone or flumazenil. Therefore, combination propofol provides the benefits of propofol-mediated sedation while reducing the risk of rapid, irreversible oversedation.[12]

The published protocols for combination propofol sedation all include a preinduction dose of either an opioid (fentanyl, 25–75 μg; meperidine, 25–50 mg), a benzodiazepine (midazolam, 0.5–2.5 mg), or both.[5,11] An induction dose of propofol then is administered (5–15 mg), followed by additional boluses of 5 to 15 mg titrated to effect. Most protocols target moderate rather than deep sedation. A nurse has primary responsibility for monitoring the patient; however, in contrast with NAPS, both the nurse and the endoscopist participate in all dosing decisions that involve propofol. Furthermore, the nurse responsible for sedation also may perform brief, interruptible tasks such as assisting with tissue acquisition. Clinical and physiologic parameters are monitored in all cases, and in some instances capnography is used as well. Several studies have reported results using a multidrug regimen. These and other studies support the observation that propofol, combined with an opioid and benzodiazepine, is an effective and safe method of sedation when administered by an endoscopist with adequate training.[11]

There is widespread belief among gastroenterologists that propofol provides better sedation for endoscopy than an opioid/benzodiazepine combination. Its benefits over traditional sedation agents are believed to include faster recovery, improved sedation effect, and greater efficiency within the endoscopy unit. Although comparative trials have shown propofol's clear-cut superiority in terms of recovery time and physician satisfaction, similar improvement in patient satisfaction has been more difficult to prove.

MEDICAL AND LEGAL IMPLICATIONS OF PROPOFOL

Although propofol has been used safely and effectively under the direction of endoscopists to provide sedation during endoscopy, the FDA-restricted product label has deterred many gastroenterologists because of concerns about potential liability for medical malpractice.[1] In most jurisdictions, FDA-approved product labels are admissible as evidence in court, so a jury would be allowed to weigh the off-label nature of gastroenterologist-directed propofol sedation. A product label alone generally is insufficient to establish the standard of care (the FDA does not regulate the practice of medicine), but it would be considered by a jury alongside expert testimony. Moreover, many jurisdictions observe the respectable minority rule, which holds that there may be multiple appropriate approaches to a particular medical problem. Numerous clinical studies, professional society guidelines, and expert editorial opinions position this as a respectable minority practice.[13] Thus, if undertaken appropriately, gastroenterologist-directed propofol sedation is reasonable from a medical and legal perspective.

Maximizing patient safety and minimizing liability when administering propofol can be accomplished by adhering to five basic principles. First, the gastroenterologist should ensure compliance with prevailing guidelines produced by professional societies as well as laws and regulations imposed by medical boards and/or credentialing bodies. Second, gastroenterologist-directed propofol sedation should be limited to appropriate, relatively low-risk patients. Third, gastroenterologists and staff should be trained in recognition and management of respiratory depression, the pharmacologic properties of propofol, and advanced cardiac life support. Fourth, endoscopy units should be equipped with resuscitation equipment and drugs, and appropriate monitoring equipment. Fifth, the informed consent discussion should inform the patient of risks, benefits, and alternatives (including the option of having propofol administered by an anesthesiologist) to gastroenterologist-directed propofol sedation, and of the qualifications and experience of the endoscopist to administer the medication. In addition, the gastroenterologist should appreciate that increased use of open-access endoscopy, in which the endoscopist may not have meaningful preprocedure contact with the patient, and increased procedure volumes may have a deleterious impact on the delivery of a thorough informed consent process.

FUTURE DIRECTIONS IN ENDOSCOPIC SEDATION

Several other innovative modalities for drug delivery to patients are being developed for endoscopic sedation. In patient-controlled analgesia/sedation (PCA/S), patient-controlled drug delivery enables the patient to control the timing of medication administration. Colonoscopy, characterized by brief periods of intense discomfort related to stretching or distension of the colon wall, would appear to be ideally suited to this method. Propofol, either alone or combined with an opioid narcotic, is the drug used most often, and multiple trials have shown that PCA/S is safe and effective for endoscopic sedation.[14,15]

On the basis of published studies, several conclusions about PCA/S and endoscopy can be drawn. First, patients receiving PCA/S experience procedure-related satisfaction that is at least comparable with, and in some cases better than, conventional sedation. Second, recovery is faster with PCA/S because the total drug dose usually is reduced. Third, PCA/S may not be suitable for all persons because it requires both the willingness and capacity to comply with instructions. Several patient characteristics have been shown to predict poor tolerance for PCA/S, including young age, female sex, and increased preprocedural anxiety.

A target-controlled infusion (TCI) system is designed to deliver an intravenous drug using an infusion pump and a computer.[16] The computer, programmed with a drug-specific, population-based pharmacokinetic model, calculates the infusion rate that is necessary to achieve the target or desired drug concentration in the blood. The computer signals the infusion pump to deliver the amount of drug necessary to achieve the predetermined drug concentration. This method of TCI, designed to deliver a target concentration of a drug that has been selected by a physician, is referred to as *open-loop* because there is no feedback from the patient. A related *closed-loop* system uses feedback from a real-time measure of drug effect such as muscle relaxation, auditory evoked potential, or another measure of sedation to regulate the concentration of delivered drug. This system should provide sedation that is more individualized, reducing the potential for undersedation and oversedation. The use of TCI, both open- and closed-loop systems, has been studied during endoscopy. The quality of sedation was considered excellent by both endoscopists and nurses. Patient satisfaction and recovery times were comparable in the two groups.[17]

Computer-assisted personalized sedation is a procedure that uses an investigational device that combines TCI of propofol and a physiologic monitoring unit.[18] The device is programmed to reduce or stop an infusion in response to either a clinical (unresponsiveness to audible/tactile stimuli) or physiologic (oxygen desaturation, hypoventilation) indication of oversedation. When patient responsiveness has returned and the physiologic parameters have been restored to normal, drug delivery is resumed at a reduced maintenance rate, based on a recalculated dosing algorithm. Computer-assisted personalized sedation is designed to deliver propofol safely and effectively when used by a trained physician/nurse team.

The feasibility of computer-assisted personalized sedation was evaluated recently by US and Belgian investigators in two studies using an identical protocol. Preliminary data suggest that computer-assisted personalized sedation may provide endoscopists with the ability to deliver propofol safely and effectively without the assistance of an anesthesia professional. A large, multicenter, pivotal trial is currently in progress.

THE ROLE OF ANESTHESIOLOGY IN CURRENT AND FUTURE GI ENDOSCOPY

The important contribution of anesthesiology in achieving satisfactory patient outcomes in current GI endoscopy is well established. The use of an anesthesia professional should be strongly considered for American Society of Anesthesiologists physical status IV and V patients or for patients undergoing emergency GI endoscopy for hemodynamically significant upper gastrointestinal bleeds. Other possible indications include children, patients with a history of alcohol or substance abuse, pregnancy, morbid obesity, neurologic or neuromuscular disorders, and patients who are uncooperative or delirious. Specific endoscopic procedures that may require an anesthesia specialist include endoscopic retrograde cholangiopancreatography (ERCP), endoscopic ultrasound, and complex, lengthy, and potentially uncomfortable therapeutic procedures such as stent placement in the upper gastrointestinal tract and esophagogastroduodenoscopy with drainage of a pseudocyst. These indications are described in detail by Goulson and Fragneto in this issue.

An additional important role for anesthesiology is in sedation quality assurance and improvement in practice safety. A system for assessing outcome measures and complications related to sedation should be established at each facility. Currently no set of clinically important quality indicators to assess adequate sedation has been accepted universally. The emphasis is instead on the documentation of sedation-related adverse events: hypoxemia requiring airway intervention, hypotension or bradycardia requiring pharmacologic intervention, pulmonary aspiration, laryngospasm, unanticipated use of reversal agents, and unanticipated hospitalization. All such adverse events as well as near misses should be reported and analyzed to identify and remedy areas of vulnerability.[19]

Digestive endoscopy has rapidly moved from being a primary diagnostic modality to being extensively used as a therapeutic modality in the management of gastrointestinal diseases. Future directions in GI endoscopy illustrate the ongoing evolution of the field as a multidisciplinary specialty combining advances in a number of areas (radiology, bioengineering, surgery, and gastroenterology). The complex nature of the following described endoscopic procedures will require the increased involvement of anesthesiology professionals to ensure successful outcomes.

NATURAL ORIFICE TRANSLUMENAL ENDOSCOPIC SURGERY

The area of most intense endoscopic investigation is natural orifice translumenal endoscopic surgery (NOTES), an amalgamation of general surgery and gastroenterology that ushers in an era of incisionless approaches to the peritoneal cavity. This term was invented during the first meeting of the Natural Orifice Surgery Consortium for Assessment and Research in July 2005.[20,21]

Currently, NOTES is performed with commercially available flexible video endoscopes, which are advanced through a natural orifice and used to create a controlled transvisceral incision that offers access to the peritoneal cavity. Once the endoscope is passed into the peritoneal cavity, endoscopic devices are advanced through the endoscope's working channels, allowing visualization and manipulation of abdominal tissues. At the completion of the procedure, the point of peritoneal access is closed using endoscopic devices, and the scope is withdrawn from the natural orifice, obviating the need for abdominal wall incisions.

The first translumenal procedures were performed in a porcine model in 2000, and multiple translumenal interventions have subsequently been completed in animal experiments and reported in abstracts and full-length articles.[21] The most common interventions include gastrojejunostomy, cholecystectomy, ligation and resection of pelvic organs, and abdominal wall hernia repair.[22] Human transgastric intraperitoneal interventions and appendectomies were initiated in India in 2003.[23] Thus far, only a limited number of human NOTES procedures have been reported in the United States, but additional translumenal human procedures have been done around the world.[23–25]

The first published human NOTES procedure described transgastric rescue of a prematurely dislodged percutaneous endoscopic gastrostomy tube.[26] The intervention started with peroral endoscopic dilation of the previous gastrostomy site by using an esophageal dilating balloon. The endoscope was then advanced through the gastrostomy into the peritoneal cavity, free fluid was aspirated from the peritoneal cavity, and a guide wire was passed through the external percutaneous endoscopic gastrostomy site into the peritoneal cavity and grasped with an endoscopic snare. The endoscope, snare, and guide wire were withdrawn into the stomach and out the mouth. The new percutaneous endoscopic gastrostomy tube was inserted over the guide wire by using the standard pull technique.

Two transvaginal, purely endoscopic appendectomies were recently reported by two independent groups of investigators from Germany and India.[23,24] Each group performed an appendectomy by using a standard flexible gastroscope and endoscopic accessories (hot biopsy forceps, needle-knives, endoclips, endoscopic detachable loops). There were no complications, and both patients recovered quickly, with an uneventful follow-up.

Other reported human NOTES interventions were done as hybrid procedures with translumenal incision and advancement of the flexible endoscope into the peritoneal cavity, along with direct laparoscopic visualization. These include two transvaginal and one transgastric appendectomies, seven transvaginal and three transgastric cholecystectomies, 10 transgastric diagnostic peritoneoscopies, and three liver biopsies.[21]

The transgastric peritoneoscopy and liver biopsies were technically simple and safe, and provided information comparable with laparoscopic abdominal exploration.[25] In addition to laparoscopic observation, the transvaginal and transgastric cholecystectomies in human beings also used laparoscopic instruments for gallbladder traction or to facilitate access to the cystic artery and cystic duct. To date no complications have been reported during or after human NOTES procedures.[23–26]

Despite the excitement that NOTES generates simply because of the novel approach it entails, sound arguments exist for its continued development. The potential advantages of NOTES approaches to peritoneal surgical issues include the elimination of skin flora–based surgical-site infections and postoperative incisional hernias, the reduction in incisional pain, and the potential for fewer intra-abdominal adhesions due to smaller access sites. The challenges that must be overcome for NOTES to become universally acceptable include reliable peritoneal access, infection prevention, suturing and anastomosis device development, user-friendly spatial orientation, multitasking platform development, intraperitoneal complication management, and reliable visceral closure. An important consideration also is the level of anesthesia that is required for specific procedures. All these principles are in the midst of intense multicenter research and development. Because NOTES occupies a medical niche that incorporates input from experts in both surgery and gastroenterology, the best training may reside in integrated training from both disciplines. This may indeed signify the end for classical training in each respective field, giving way to one hybridized field of endoscopic surgery.

SPYGLASS DIRECT PANCREATICOBILIARY VISUALIZATION SYSTEM

The SpyGlass direct visualization system (Boston Scientific, Natick, Massachusetts) is a mother–daughter scope system using a standard duodenoscope, a 10-Fr daughter scope/catheter with a 1.2-mm working channel, and a 0.77-mm-diameter fiber optic probe intended to provide direct visualization for diagnostic and therapeutic applications during endoscopic procedures in the pancreaticobiliary system, including the hepatic ducts, to identify stones and strictures.[27,28] Conventional ERCP is conducted by using two-dimensional black-and-white images rendered by fluoroscopy, which can potentially lead to an inaccurate or inconclusive clinical diagnosis, potentially creating the need for additional testing. In early trials using an animal model, the SpyGlass system was effective for access, direct visualization, and biopsy in all bile duct quadrants. In addition, SpyGlass procedures can be performed by a single operator, unlike conventional therapeutic upper endoscopy, which requires an operator and an assistant.

The cholangioscopy procedure with the SpyGlass system is performed with the access-and-delivery catheter positioned just below the operating channel of the duodenoscope. The duodenoscope is positioned in front of the papilla, and a sphincterotomy is performed as necessary. The SpyGlass system is introduced into the therapeutic duodenoscope. The bile duct is cannulated, and the SpyScope catheter is used to guide the SpyGlass visualization probe into the biliary tree. The SpyScope catheter and SpyGlass probe are maneuvered up to the desired area of interest within the duct for direct visualization. In addition, selected ducts and branches of interest can be examined during repeated advancement and withdrawal of the system. A Spy-Bite biopsy forceps guided by using the SpyScope catheter can be introduced, and an endoscopically guided biopsy can be performed. Also, electrohydraulic lithotripsy can be used as needed via a 3-Fr electrohydraulic lithotripsy probe passed through the 1.2-mm working channel. Once this is completed, a standard stone retrieval basket or balloon is used to clear the duct of any remaining stone fragments.[27,28]

A recent case series compared results of conventional ERCP and single-operator duodenoscope-assisted cholangiopancreatoscopy using the SpyGlass direct visualization system. Direct visualization with SpyGlass altered the clinicians' diagnosis or treatment strategy for 19 of 22 patients who had previously been examined unsuccessfully using ERCP but suspected of harboring malignancy, bile duct strictures, retained bile duct stones, or cystic biliary lesions. Overall, SpyGlass examination with or without biopsy was accomplished without technical difficulty for 20 of the 22 cases.[27,28]

This novel technology now allows direct optical diagnostic and therapeutic means where previously only indirect radiographic imaging was available for intervention guidance. The potential applicability of this technology is expanding as other regions in the human body currently too remote or fragile for standard instrument navigation are being investigated.[29]

BARRX MEDICAL HALO SYSTEM

The HALO system (both HALO 360 and HALO 90; BARRX Medical, Inc., Sunnyvale, California), is a novel device designed to treat and circumferentially ablate the esophageal mucosa of patients who have Barrett's esophagus without harming the underlying tissue layers. Cleared by the US FDA in 2001, the HALO system has been commercially available since January 2005.

Using standard endoscopic techniques with the patient under conscious sedation, the HALO system facilitates rapid ablation of long and short segments of Barrett's esophagus in three steps. Initially, the anatomic landmarks and length of Barrett's epithelium are identified by esophagoscopy. A sizing balloon then is used to measure the inner diameter of the esophagus and select the appropriately sized ablation catheter. Finally, a radiofrequency ablation catheter is deployed, which circumferentially ablates a 3-cm-long segment of Barrett's epithelium in less than 1 second. A consistent ablation depth of less than 1 mm avoids damage to the submucosal tissue layers.[30]

Two recent studies established that use of the HALO system was safe and effective for the treatment of patients with Barrett's esophagus and low- or high-grade dysplasia.[30,31] After two treatment sessions, 10 of 11 patients had a complete response for dysplasia. The patient with persistent dysplasia went from high- to low-grade dysplasia and had only small residual islands of Barrett's mucosa left. In the same patient group, the internal esophageal diameter was identical before treatment and 10 weeks afterward, confirming that radiofrequency ablation, in contrast to other ablative and resective techniques, does not result in significant scarring or structuring. In the largest clinical trial of the HALO system to date, the average procedure time was less than 30 minutes. At the 1-year follow-up assessment, 70% of the patients were free of Barrett's esophagus, and no strictures or buried glands were detected in 3,007 surveillance biopsies.[30–32]

ENDOSCOPIC MUCOSAL RESECTION/ENDOSCOPIC SUBMUCOSAL DISSECTION

Endoscopic mucosal resection has been incorporated in Asia as a curative treatment for superficial carcinomas in the foregut. The technique incorporates accessing mucosal lesions via an endoscope, splitting the mucosal/submucosal plane of a segment of the gastrointestinal tract, and removing the mucosal lesion while preserving the submucosa and adventitia of the hollow viscus. Experience with this technique in Western Europe and the Americas is limited because of infrequent screening and diagnosis of early gastric cancers, compared with Japanese and Korean populations.

The use of endoscopic mucosal resection, however, is increasing outside Asia. Deprez and colleagues[33] describe recent results for more than 170 Belgian patients managed satisfactorily with endoscopic resection of esophageal high-grade dysplasia or squamous cell carcinoma and gastric or Barrett's epithelium high-grade dysplasia or adenocarcinoma. Similar results were seen by Ross and colleagues,[34] who treated 16 patients between 2003 and 2005. Of the patients staged as being T1aN0Mx using pretreatment endoscopic ultrasound and found to have corresponding histopathology, none experienced recurrence at a median follow-up assessment 17 months after treatment, according to surveillance endoscopic biopsies. Ell and colleagues[35] recently reported complete local remission for 99 of 100 patients who underwent endoscopic mucosal resection for mucosally based early esophageal adenocarcinoma. Although 11% experienced recurrent or metachronous lesions in the 3 years after treatment, all of these patients were treated successfully with repeat endoscopic resection.

Innovative devices have furthered this relatively young technology, and Seewald and colleagues[36] describe their initial experience with the newly introduced Duette Multiband Mucosectomy Kit (Cook Ireland Ltd, Limerick, Ireland) for the treatment of extensive early esophageal squamous cell carcinoma. The device allows for repeated ligation and resection of targeted mucosal regions without removal and reinsertion of the endoscope. Five patients with more than hemicircumferential involvement of the esophageal wall and a mean involved length of 2.8 cm were successfully treated in one session using endoscopic mucosal resection. Posttreatment stricture was successfully treated using bougienage, and no recurrences were noted 1 year after treatment.

In addition, a modified rigid endoscopic device for suction resection of mucosal lesions (Karl Storz GmbH, Tuttlingen, Germany) is being introduced. This device operates by suctioning a large mucosal area against a transparent and perforated hemicylindrical window. Mucosal resection is performed by using an electrical wire loop at a constant depth of 1 mm. Jaquet and colleagues[37] performed endoscopic mucosal resection in a series of animal trials using hemicircumferential and circumferential mucosectomies 2 to 6 cm long. The deep resection margin of the specimens was noted to be located precisely at the submucosal level.

Despite the seemingly straightforward objectives of endoscopic mucosal resection, difficulty in correctly assessing the depth of tumor invasion and an increase in local recurrence have been reported in cases of large lesions because such lesions often are resected piecemeal. An innovation on standard endoscopic mucosal resection termed *endoscopic submucosal dissection* allows direct dissection of the submucosa and en bloc resection of large lesions. Endoscopic submucosal dissection is not limited by resection size, however. It still is associated with a higher incidence of complications than endoscopic mucosal resection and requires a high level of endoscopic skill.[38]

Endoscopic submucosal dissection allows for the same approach as that used for mucosal resection, except that the deeper submucosal tissue plane is opened with the aid of tissue elevation using solutions such as saline, glycerol, sodium hyaluronate, or fructose immediately before the dissection. Although technically demanding, endoscopic submucosal dissection is quite effective. Imagawa and colleagues[39] report an 84% rate of curative en bloc resection from 2002 through 2005. The perforation rate was 6%, and each perforation was managed endoscopically. No local recurrences were observed among the 119 curatively resected lesions 1 year after dissection. This technique has even been applied successfully to patients who have undergone insufficient previous endoscopic mucosal resection. Oka and colleagues[40] report successful dissection and resection in 14 of 15 patients who had residual disease after mucosal resection. No recurrences were noted during a mean follow-up period of 18 months. Currently, this technique is being evaluated for the resection of gastric subepithelial tumors from the muscularis propria, including gastrointestinal stromal tumors. Lee and colleagues[41] report the successful excision of 9 in 12 applicable lesions in 11 patients between 2004 and 2006. No patients experienced perforation or hemorrhage.

HIGH-RESOLUTION AND MAGNIFICATION ENDOSCOPY, AND CHROMOENDOSCOPY

To identify lesions amenable for the BARRX Halo system, endoscopic mucosal resection, and endoscopic submucosal dissection treatment modalities, advances had to be made in endoscopic imaging abilities. Conventional endoscopy is characterized by resolution of from 100,000 to 300,000 pixels. Subsequent generations of endoscopic techniques require cameras of 400,000, even 850,000, pixels that are referred to as *high resolution endoscopes*. These endoscopes are equipped with optic zoom composed of movable motor-driven lens. Changing the focus of the lens provides considerable magnification of the observed area, of from 80 to 200 times. It is used in diagnosis of subtle mucosal abnormalities of 1 to 2 mm in diameter to detect early cancerous changes and to direct the precise biopsy of pathological changes.[42,43]

Chromoendoscopy technique uses a locally staining agent applied to the mucous membrane during endoscopy to characterize the changes better. It has become useful in early diagnosis of malignancies and other nonneoplastic conditions. The method is cheap, the coloring agents are widely accessible and nontoxic, and there are no side effects noted if they are used in small, recommended quantities.

Chromoendoscopy became more important when magnifying and high-resolution endoscopy methods were introduced.[44,45] Contrast chromoendoscopy that colors the mucous depressions uses from 1 to 25 mL of 0.1% to 1% solution of indigo carmine (blue pigment), depending on the size of the area examined. The mucosa is examined immediately after the stain has been administered. The method is used to detect early cancers of the esophagus, stomach, and colon, to diagnose Barrett's esophagus, to assess villous atrophy of the intestine, and to detect discrete mucosal loss.[46,47]

Different coloring agents that are absorbed by certain type of cells are used in absorptive staining. Lugol's solution (a dark-brown staining agent) stains glycogen-rich cells of the esophageal epithelium. Following administration, normal, smooth, nonkeratinized esophageal epithelium turns dark brown or green-brown. No change in color suggests abnormal epithelium such as erosive esophagitis, and cancerous metaplastic or dysplastic foci. The inability to differentiate between different conditions requires repeated biopsies of the changed mucosa. Methylene blue 0.2% is a blue staining agent that is actively absorbed by epithelial cells of the small and large intestine. Toluidine blue accumulates in dysplastic and atypical cells with increased DNA proliferation. Toluidine blue stains dysplastic and neoplastic, but not benign, cells dark blue or dark purple-blue. Other staining agents used in absorptive chromoendoscopy are cresyl violet, which diffuses into mucosal depressions, and crystal violet, which stains intestinal metaplastic foci. Absorptive chromoendoscopy is used to diagnose early stages of esophageal cancer and Barrett's esophagus, to locate intestinal metaplastic foci inside the stomach, to identify ectopic gastric mucosa in the duodenum, and to detect colon adenomas and adenocarcinoma.[48] Application of these different stains lengthen the duration of endoscopic procedures considerably, necessitating increased attention to sedation requirements.

DEEP-BALLOON ENTEROSCOPY

Videoenteroscopy is a new endoscopic visualization technique of the small intestine. It was designed by Yamamoto and colleagues in 2001.[49] A typical double-balloon enteroscope is composed of a 200-cm-long endoscope, a 145-cm-long semielastic external tube, and two latex balloons to better fix the endoscope inside the small intestine and for easier penetration. The endoscope can be inserted via the stomach or can be used to approach from the ileocecal valve. The choice of the route depends on the expected localization of the pathology. If the examination of the entire small intestine is required, both routes of insertion should be used after the farthest destination point has been marked with a submucosal marker during the first examination. When the marked point has been reached during subsequent examination using the other route, it implies that the entire length of the small intestine had been examined. Double- and single-balloon techniques, as well as spiral enteroscopy techniques, have been described. The examination of the entire small intestine generally requires more than 2 hours on average, with an increased need for sedation and anesthesiology input. The technique is 80% to 90% effective and failure is most often due to postoperative adhesions.[50] Deep-balloon enteroscopy is recommended in the evaluation of Crohn's disease involving the small bowel, identification of a bleeding source, detection of stenoses and neoplastic changes in the small intestine, and investigation of obscure causes of chronic diarrhea and malabsorption syndromes.[51] Few complications have been described, such as pancreatitis and perforation or microperforation of the small intestine, all of which were treated conservatively.[52,53] In addition to diagnostic possibilities, enteroscopy allows both biopsy of affected areas and endoscopic therapy. The double-balloon enteroscopy method has been the best described and is now considered the "gold standard" in the diagnosis and endoscopic treatment of small intestine diseases. The increased duration of the examination, the sedation requirements, and the use of fluoroscopy may pose some limitations to the procedure.

SUMMARY

A successful population-based colorectal cancer screening requires efficient colonoscopy practices that incorporate high throughput, safety, and patient satisfaction. There are several different modalities of nonanesthesiologist-administered sedation currently available and in development that may fulfill these requirements. Modern-day gastroenterology endoscopic procedures are complex and demand the full attention of the attending gastroenterologist and the complete cooperation of the patient. Many of these procedures will also require the anesthesiologist's knowledge, skills, abilities, and experience to ensure optimal procedure results and good patient outcomes.

REFERENCES

1. Cohen LB, Wecsler JS, Gaetano JN, et al. Endoscopic sedation in the United States: results from a nationwide survey. Am J Gastroenterol 2006;101:967–74.
2. Huang YY, Lee HK, Juan CH, et al. Conscious sedation in gastrointestinal endoscopy. Acta Anaesthesiol Taiwan 2005;43:33–8.
3. Cohen LB, Delegge MH, Aisenberg J, et al. AGA Institute review of endoscopic sedation. Gastroenterology 2007;133:675–701.
4. Byrne MF, Baillie J. Nurse-assisted propofol sedation: the jury is in!. Gastroenterology 2005;129:1781–2.
5. Clarke AC, Chiragakis L, Hillman LC, et al. Sedation for endoscopy: the safe use of propofol by general practitioner sedationists. Med J Aust 2002;176:158–61.
6. Heuss LT, Schnieper P, Drewe J, et al. Safety of propofol for conscious sedation during endoscopic procedures in high-risk patients—a prospective, controlled study. Am J Gastroenterol 2003;98:1751–7.
7. Rex DK, Heuss LT, Walker JA, et al. Trained registered nurses/endoscopy teams can administer propofol safely for endoscopy. Gastroenterology 2005;129:1384–91.
8. Aisenberg J, Brill JV, Ladabaum U, et al. Sedation for gastrointestinal endoscopy: new practices, new economics. Am J Gastroenterol 2005;100:996–1000.
9. Rex DK. The science and politics of propofol. Am J Gastroenterol 2004;99:2080–3.
10. Tohda G, Higashi S, Wakahara S, et al. Propofol sedation during endoscopic procedures: safe and effective administration by registered nurses supervised by endoscopists. Endoscopy 2006;38:360–7.
11. Cohen LB, Dubovsky AN, Aisenberg J, et al. Propofol for endoscopic sedation: a protocol for safe and effective administration by the gastroenterologist. Gastrointest Endosc 2003;58:725–32.
12. Cohen LB, Hightower CD, Wood DA, et al. Moderate level sedation during endoscopy: a prospective study using low-dose propofol, meperidine/fentanyl, and midazolam. Gastrointest Endosc 2004;59:795–803.
13. Aisenberg J, Cohen LB, Piorkowski JD Jr. Propofol use under the direction of trained gastroenterologists: an analysis of the medicolegal implications. Am J Gastroenterol 2007;102:707–13.
14. Heuss LT, Drewe J, Schnieper P, et al. Patient-controlled versus nurse-administered sedation with propofol during colonoscopy. A prospective randomized trial. Am J Gastroenterol 2004;99:511–8.
15. Lee DW, Chan AC, Wong SK, et al. The safety, feasibility, and acceptability of patient-controlled sedation for colonoscopy: prospective study. Hong Kong Med J 2004;10:84–8.
16. Egan TD. Target-controlled drug delivery: progress toward an intravenous "vaporizer" and automated anesthetic administration. Anesthesiology 2003;99:1214–9.
17. Fanti L, Agostoni M, Casati A, et al. Target-controlled propofol infusion during monitored anesthesia in patients undergoing ERCP. Gastrointest Endosc 2004;60:361–6.
18. Doufas AG, Bakhshandeh M, Bjorksten AR, et al. Induction speed is not a determinant of propofol pharmacodynamics. Anesthesiology 2004;101:1112–21.
19. American Society for Gastrointestinal Endoscopy. Guidelines for training in patient monitoring and sedation and analgesia. Gastrointest Endosc 1998;48:669–71.

20. Rattner D. Introduction to NOTES White Paper. Surg Endosc 2006;20:185.
21. Rattner D, Kalloo A. ASGE/SAGES Working Group on Natural Orifice Translume-nal Endoscopic Surgery. 2005. Surg Endosc 2006;20:329–33.
22. Mintz Y, Horgan S, Cullen J, et al. NOTES: the hybrid technique. J Laparoendosc Adv Surg Tech A 2007;17:402–6.
23. Palanivelu C, Rajan PS, Rangarajan M, et al. Transvaginal endoscopic appendec-tomy in humans: a unique approach to NOTES—world's first report. Surg Endosc 2008. [Epub ahead of print].
24. Bernhardt J, Gerber B, Schober HC, et al. NOTES—case report of a unidirectional flexible appendectomy. Int J Colorectal Dis 2008;23:547–50.
25. Steele K, Schweitzer MA, Lyn-Sue J, et al. Flexible transgastric peritoneoscopy and liver biopsy: a feasibility study in human beings (with videos). Gastrointest Endosc 2008;68:61–6.
26. Marks JM, Ponsky JL, Pearl JP, et al. PEG "Rescue": a practical NOTES technique. Surg Endosc 2007;21:816–9.
27. Chen YK. Preclinical characterization of the Spyglass peroral cholangiopancrea-toscopy system for direct access, visualization, and biopsy. Gastrointest Endosc 2007;65:303–11.
28. Chen YK, Pleskow DK. SpyGlass single-operator peroral cholangiopancreato-scopy system for the diagnosis and therapy of bile-duct disorders: a clinical feasibility study (with video). Gastrointest Endosc 2007;65:832–41.
29. Antillon MR, Tiwari P, Bartalos CR, et al. Taking SpyGlass outside the GI tract lumen in conjunction with EUS to assist in the diagnosis of a pancreatic cystic lesion (with video). Gastrointest Endosc 2008. [Epub ahead of print].
30. Dunkin BJ, Martinez J, Bejarano PA, et al. Thin-layer ablation of human esopha-geal epithelium using a bipolar radiofrequency balloon device. Surg Endosc 2006;20:125–30.
31. Bergman JJ. Radiofrequency energy ablation of Barrett's esophagus: the best is yet to come!. Gastrointest Endosc 2007;65:200–2.
32. Bergman JJ. Endoscopic resection for treatment of mucosal Barrett's cancer: time to swing the pendulum. Gastrointest Endosc 2007;65:11–3.
33. Deprez PH, Aouattah T, Piessevaux H. Endoscopic removal or ablation of oesophageal and gastric superficial tumours. Acta Gastroenterol Belg 2006;69:304–11.
34. Ross AS, Noffsinger A, Waxman I. Narrow band imaging directed EMR for Barrett's esophagus with high-grade dysplasia. Gastrointest Endosc 2007;65:166–9.
35. Ell C, May A, Pech O, et al. Curative endoscopic resection of early esophageal adenocarcinomas (Barrett's cancer). Gastrointest Endosc 2007;65:3–10.
36. Seewald S, Ang TL, Omar S, et al. Endoscopic mucosal resection of early esoph-ageal squamous cell cancer using the Duette mucosectomy kit. Endoscopy 2006;38:1029–31.
37. Jaquet Y, Pilloud R, Grosjean P, et al. Extended endoscopic mucosal resection in the esophagus and hypopharynx: a new rigid device. Eur Arch Otorhinolaryngol 2007;264:57–62.
38. Gotoda T, Yamamoto H, Soetikno RM. Endoscopic submucosal dissection of early gastric cancer. J Gastroenterol 2006;41:929–42.
39. Imagawa A, Okada H, Kawahara Y, et al. Endoscopic submucosal dissection for early gastric cancer: results and degrees of technical difficulty as well as success. Endoscopy 2006;38:987–90.
40. Oka S, Tanaka S, Kaneko I, et al. Endoscopic submucosal dissection for residual/local recurrence of early gastric cancer after endoscopic mucosal resection. Endoscopy 2006;38:996–1000.

41. Lee IL, Lin PY, Tung SY, et al. Endoscopic submucosal dissection for the treatment of intraluminal gastric subepithelial tumors originating from the muscularis propria layer. Endoscopy 2006;38:1024–8.
42. Nelson DB, Block KP, Bosco JJ, et al. High resolution and high-magnification endoscopy: September 2000. Gastrointest Endosc 2000;52:864–6.
43. Skrzypek T, Valverde Piedra JL, Skrzypek H, et al. Light and scanning electron microscopy evaluation of the postnatal small intestinal mucosa development in pigs. J Physiol Pharmacol 2005;56(Suppl 3):71–87.
44. Acosta MM, Boyce HW Jr. Chromoendoscopy—where is it useful? J Clin Gastroenterol 1998;27:13–20.
45. Fennerty MB. Tissue staining (chromoscopy) of the gastrointestinal tract. Can J Gastroenterol 1999;13:423–9.
46. Kiesslich R, Mergener K, Naumann C, et al. Value of chromoendoscopy and magnification endoscopy in the evaluation of duodenal abnormalities: a prospective, randomized comparison. Endoscopy 2003;35:559–63.
47. Stevens PD, Lightdale CJ, Green PH, et al. Combined magnification endoscopy with chromoendoscopy for the evaluation of Barrett's esophagus. Gastrointest Endosc 1994;40:747–9.
48. Tabuchi M, Sueoka N, Fujimori T. Videoendoscopy with vital double dye staining (crystal violet and methylene blue) for detection of a minute focus of early stage adenocarcinoma in Barrett's esophagus: a case report. Gastrointest Endosc 2001;54:385–8.
49. Yamamoto H, Sekine Y, Sato Y, et al. Total enteroscopy with a nonsurgical steerable double-balloon method. Gastrointest Endosc 2001;53:216–20.
50. May A, Nachbar L, Schneider M, et al. Push-and-pull enteroscopy using the double-balloon technique: method of assessing depth of insertion and training of the enteroscopy technique using the Erlangen Endo-Trainer. Endoscopy 2005;37:66–70.
51. May A, Nachbar L, Ell C. Double-balloon enteroscopy (push-and-pull enteroscopy) of the small bowel: feasibility and diagnostic and therapeutic yield in patients with suspected small bowel disease. Gastrointest Endosc 2005;62: 62–70.
52. Mensink PB, Haringsma J, Kucharzik T, et al. Complications of double balloon enteroscopy: a multicenter survey. Endoscopy 2007;39:613–5.
53. Yamamoto H, Kita H, Sunada K, et al. Clinical outcomes of double-balloon endoscopy for the diagnosis and treatment of small-intestinal diseases. Clin Gastroenterol Hepatol 2004;2:1010–6.

Interventional Radiology and Anesthesia

Matthew P. Schenker, MD[a], Ramon Martin, MD[b],
Paul B. Shyn, MD[c], Richard A. Baum, MD[a],*

KEYWORDS

- Anesthesia • Interventional radiology • Quality assurance
- Sedation • Angiography

During the past the decade interventional radiology (IR) has evolved from a referral-based to a clinically based specialty. Longitudinal care now is provided to patients before, during, and after procedures. This paradigm shift has resulted in dramatic increases in the scope and volume of practice and in the complexity of patients undergoing image-guided procedures.

The need for anesthesia and procedural sedation outside the operating room (OR) continues to grow as the number of minimally invasive procedures proliferates and the complexity of cases undertaken outside the OR increases. The division of Angiography and Interventional Radiology at Brigham and Women's Hospital has witnessed a greater than fourfold increase in the number of cases requiring procedural sedation during the 5-year period ending in April 2008, with a concomitant growth in the number of cases requiring monitored anesthesia care (MAC) or general anesthesia (GA). This trend is likely to accelerate as the population ages and minimally invasive procedures continue to supplement or replace traditional open surgeries.

How are medical specialists to address this burgeoning need for procedural sedation in a safe and effective manner? Anesthesiologists are well equipped to deliver anesthesia and procedural sedation by virtue of their specialty training and broad experience in a number of settings. These settings include the OR, emergency

This article originally appeared in *Anesthesiology Clinics of North America*, Volume 27, Issue 1.
[a] Division of Angiography and Interventional Radiology, Department of Radiology, Brigham and Women's Hospital, Harvard Medical School, 75 Francis Street, Boston, MA 02115, USA
[b] Department of Anesthesiology, Perioperative and Pain Medicine, Brigham and Women's Hospital, Harvard Medical School, 75 Francis Street, Boston, MA 02115, USA
[c] Division of Abdominal Imaging and Intervention, Department of Radiology, Brigham and Women's Hospital, Harvard Medical School, 75 Francis Street, Boston, MA 02115, USA
* Corresponding author. Division of Angiography and Interventional Radiology, Department of Radiology, Brigham and Women's Hospital, Harvard Medical School, 75 Francis Street, Boston, MA 02115.
E-mail address: rbaum@partners.org (R.A. Baum).

Perioperative Nursing Clinics 4 (2009) 451–458
doi:10.1016/j.cpen.2009.09.010
1556-7931/09/$ – see front matter © 2009 Elsevier Inc. All rights reserved.

room, ICU, pain clinic, and other procedural areas. The availability of anesthesiologists will become more limited as the demand for their expertise grows. How, then, can this expert resource be used effectively to maximize patient comfort and safety during diagnostic and therapeutic procedures? This article illustrates how these policies and procedures have evolved at Brigham and Women's Hospital and in the authors' division with the goals of delineating the important components of a proficient model for collaboration with the anesthesia staff and identifying future challenges facing all providers who are involved in minimally invasive procedures.

The OR model of anesthesia care is extended to procedures in the IR suite. The model of care includes

1. Adequate preprocedural assessment to determine the patient's need for anesthesia care during the procedure
2. Standardized monitoring and anesthesia equipment
3. Clearly marked and easily accessible emergency equipment (code cart, defibrillator)
4. Adequate back-up in case of emergencies or difficulties
5. Postoperative care in a postanesthesia care unit setting

With an increasing array of imaging techniques and instruments, interventional radiologists now perform procedures that once were surgical and main OR staples. In addition to regularly scheduled procedures that may require general anesthesia (ablation of venous and arteriovenous malformations, aortic endoleak repair, complex vascular stenting procedures, among others), there also are an array of emergent procedures (embolization for upper or lower gastrointestinal bleeding, hemoptysis, trauma, postpartum hemorrhage or percutaneous drainage for urosepsis and biliary sepsis, among others) that come first to the IR suite and then to the OR if necessary. These cases all require intense anesthesia care despite their minimally invasive character and non-OR venue (**Box 1**).

The difficulties inherent in IR suite procedures relate to both the technical intricacies of the procedures and the comorbidities of the patients. Interventional radiologists are relied upon to perform highly targeted, technically demanding interventions in the safest and most efficient manner for their patients. Often, interventional radiologists are asked to treat patients who cannot physically tolerate an alternative open surgery. IR treatment, however, does not mean that these "nonsurgical" candidates will not require MAC or GA for their minimally invasive procedures, a common misconception among surgical specialists who refer their patients to IR. It also does not mean that the procedure is less risky because it is not "open."

It is, therefore, increasingly common for an interventional radiologist ask the consulting anesthesiologist to assess the overall clinical picture of such "nonsurgical" candidates to devise an anesthesia care plan for the IR procedure. Assessments of a patient's body habitus and condition, underlying cardiopulmonary status, oncologic

---

Box 1
Non–operating room locations for radiology/anesthesia

Angiography and interventional radiology

CT

MRI

Interventional neuroradiology

and other medical history, and various psychosocial issues are critical to both the anesthesia care of these patients and the outcome of the procedure. The determination of the best anesthesia plan is a function of the patient's medical condition and the details of the IR procedure and, therefore, requires direct and frequent communication between the anesthesiologist and interventional radiologist.

The following discussion considers some angiographic and cross-sectional IR procedures in more detail and comments on some of the anesthesia choices and considerations. In addition, specific concerns and conflicts in the area of IR are mentioned.

ANGIOGRAPHY AND INTERVENTIONAL RADIOLOGY

The practice of angiography and IR encompasses a wide range of procedures on many different organ systems. Approximately 70% of the procedures performed are booked less than 48 hours in advance because of the relatively urgent or emergent nature of the bulk of IR procedures. Even though most of these procedures are done with a nurse providing moderate sedation and analgesia, there is a continual discussion between the anesthesia and IR staff about how best to provide for patient comfort and safety. An accurate and complete preprocedural assessment is key to having a patient comfortably tolerate a procedure (ie, hold still, breathe, and experience no pain). As a result, a member of the anesthesia team is involved in evaluating patients in far more than the 10% of IR cases that actually require MAC or GA.

Most IR procedures require that the patient lie supine. Pain from arthritis and surgical incisions, respiratory compromise from chronic obstructive pulmonary disease, pneumonia, pleural effusions, obstructive sleep apnea, and inability to cooperate because of dementia or language differences can make a seemingly straightforward procedure, such as placement of a portacath or tunneled catheter a very difficult problem in terms of the sedation plan. Some procedures, such as emergent transjugular portosystemic shunt creation, deep tissue sclerotherapy, placement of a translumbar dialysis catheter, or embolization for hemorrhage in hypotensive patients, present clear-cut choices for anesthesia care. Other procedures, such as percutaneous nephrostomies, biliary drainage, dialysis shunt maintenance, and major vessel stenting involve little discomfort after the placement of the initial access, but the patient must lie still and be able to cooperate when asked. In such situations, patient comorbidities can influence the choice of sedation and analgesia.

CROSS-SECTIONAL INTERVENTIONAL RADIOLOGY

Cross-sectional imaging modalities, including computed tomography (CT), magnetic resonance imaging (MRI), and ultrasound (US), are used to guide a variety of interventional procedures performed by interventional radiologists. The most common procedures are percutaneous biopsies, aspirations, and drainages performed in almost any body region. Many other interventional procedures, including cyst or tumor ablations, nerve blocks, and pseudoaneurysm occlusions, are performed with cross-sectional imaging guidance.

CT- and US-guided interventional procedures range from easily and quickly performed procedures requiring minimal patient cooperation and sedation to prolonged, difficult procedures necessitating patient cooperation or careful control of breathing along with significant pain control. Respiratory parameters are critical to many of these procedures because of the changes induced in target location and anatomic morphology. Respiratory motion is most problematic in procedures involving structures near the diaphragm, such as liver, adrenals, kidneys, and the lower half of the lungs. A helpful strategy in many of these procedures is to begin sedation early so that by the time initial planning scans are obtained, the patient is sedated and respirations have become shallower with reduced tidal volume. Such an approach increases the likelihood of selecting an optimal skin entry site for the percutaneous procedure.

Pain from needle biopsies varies with anatomic site and depth of needle penetration. In general, however, the level of sedation required is relatively constant throughout the needle placement and imaging phases of the procedure. With percutaneous catheter drainages, the level of pain control required tends to increase progressively from the initial needle placement through the track dilation steps and to the final catheter placement.

Percutaneous ethanol ablation is indicated for symptomatic, recurrent cysts in the liver or kidney. The initial needle placement and small-diameter catheter placement, often 6 F, usually is well tolerated, but the actual ethanol injection can produce considerable pain. Communication and coordination between the interventional radiologist and anesthesiologist therefore is needed.

Increasingly, percutaneous tumor ablation procedures are performed to manage malignant lesions throughout the body but most commonly in the liver, kidney, adrenals, lung, or bone. A variety of technologies are used, including radiofrequency ablation, cryoablation, microwave ablation, and ethanol ablation, among others. Although some ablation procedures are completed easily in less than 1 hour, completion of other cases may require up to 3 or 4 hours.

These procedures may require the precise placement of five or more needle probes into the target organ or tissue. Some radiofrequency ablation devices allow placement of a single needle probe with the subsequent deployment of an expandable array of tynes or electrodes into the target area. Other radiofrequency devices and cryoablation probes may require placement of multiple needle probes. Radiofrequency ablation accomplishes tumor destruction through tissue heating, whereas cryoablation accomplishes tumor destruction through freezing. Freezing of tissues with cryoablation tends to cause less pain than heating with radiofrequency ablation.

Regardless of the ablation technology used, reproducible levels of breath holding often are important in facilitating optimal and safe probe placements. This breath holding can be accomplished either with a degree of conscious sedation that allows good patient cooperation or with general anesthesia and same-level interruption of ventilation.

A specific problem encountered in ablation procedures of adrenal tumors or tumors adjacent to the adrenal gland is catecholamine-induced hypertensive crisis. This problem is most likely to occur when residual normal adrenal tissue is present and is less likely to occur when the adrenal is replaced completely by tumor. Radiofrequency ablation tends to stimulate catecholamine release during the application of heat to the adrenal tissue. With cryoablation, on the other hand, catecholamine release is not observed during the freeze but instead occurs during or following the thaw phase. Pharmacologic pretreatment strategies may be considered but do not necessarily prevent such hypertensive crises.

An increasingly popular CT-guided ablation procedure in the pediatric population is radiofrequency ablation of benign osteoid osteomas of bone. These painful bone lesions often are cured with percutaneous ablation, thus avoiding an open surgical procedure. Because of patient age and the significant pain associated with heating these lesions typically located adjacent to the periosteum, general anesthesia often is preferred.

MRI is not commonly used to guide IR procedures because of the many technical challenges involved in operating in an environment with a strong magnetic field. Nevertheless, the advantages of MRI, including superior soft tissue contrast, multiplanar imaging capabilities, and lack of ionizing radiation, probably will drive the increasing use of MRI for select interventional procedures. MRI guidance is favored for biopsies or ablations of target lesions not well visualized on CT or US imaging.

Positron emission tomography (PET)/CT also will be increasingly useful in guiding IR procedures when the metabolic characteristics of target lesions can be exploited for targeting purposes. The challenges of PET/CT-guided interventions include image-acquisition times of up to several minutes within a long scanner gantry and potential radiation exposure to operating personnel from high-energy radiopharmaceuticals.

As the scope and complexity of cross-sectional IR procedures continue to grow, the need for a reliable interface with anesthesiologists is clear. The use of more sophisticated sedation techniques and the formulation or supervision of an anesthetic plan of care, whether it be deep sedation or general anesthesia, is becoming increasingly important to the efficiency and success of new cross-sectional IR procedures.

ANESTHESIOLOGISTS IN INTERVENTIONAL RADIOLOGY

The unanticipated need for anesthesia support during a procedure can compromise patient safety and affect the success of the procedure. Effort therefore is focused on preprocedural patient screening. When patients who have potentially problematic comorbidities present for an elective procedure, they are sent to the preadmitting testing center for a complete assessment and are booked for their procedure with an anesthesiologist. Although this approach is time consuming, it is far preferable to a failed attempt at performing the procedure under moderate sedation alone, without an anesthesiologist present. The latter scenario creates the potential need to reschedule the case or, worse, requires an anesthesia urgent consultation or intervention while the patient is on the table in distress.

For non-elective or emergent procedures, the interventional radiologist is responsible for informing the anesthesiologist about the complexity and anticipated duration of the procedure and whether MAC or GA may be required. Anesthesiologists assigned to IR must make a crucial determination whenever they are asked to evaluate a patient for procedural sedation, namely, are there comorbid conditions that preclude the safe administration of moderate procedural sedation and analgesia by a non–anesthesia provider?

Preprocedure patient assessment in IR can be extremely time consuming and may become impossible for one individual anesthesiologist manage. Because of the increasing case load in IR and the inability to capture all relevant aspects of the patient's history, the authors use a nurse practitioner to assist with new patient evaluations in the IR suite. These evaluations include everything from routine airway evaluations to comprehensive history and physicals for more complicated patients. The nurse practitioner acts as an important intermediary between the anesthesia and IR staff. This approach allows more timely patient evaluations, emphasizing both the airway examination and, more importantly, the patient's overall clinical status. It has helped expedite the implementation of required treatments by both the interventional radiologists and the anesthesiologists.

Although preprocedure assessment is crucial, interventional radiologists also rely on the advice and direction of their anesthesia colleagues on how to perform moderate sedation in the safest possible manner and how to certify the providers who are responsible for its administration. The authors reference the revised practice guidelines published by the American Society of Anesthesiologists in 2002 for sedation and analgesia by non-anesthesiologists. This revision includes two important changes from previous editions: (1) it defines "deep sedation" as distinct from moderate or "conscious" sedation because of the greater likelihood that deep sedation could inadvertently progress to general anesthesia, and (2) it recommends that all practitioners administering sedation possess the ability to rescue patients from profound sedation or some complication thereof.[1] To fulfill these requirements, every physician and nurse in the Department of Radiology is required to maintain biennial certification in advanced cardiac life support (ACLS). They also are required to maintain biennial certification in moderate sedation and analgesia, also known as "intravenous conscious sedation." This dedicated training course emphasizes the pharmacology of agents commonly used during sedation and the antagonists used for the reversal of sedation.

IMPACT OF THE ENVIRONMENT

Nearly half the anesthesia claims reviewed by Bhanakor and colleagues[2] could have been prevented by better monitoring or improved vigilance. The most common potential mechanism for patient injury during procedural sedation is respiratory depression caused by an overdose of sedative drugs. Proper monitoring equipment is essential whenever and wherever procedural sedation is administered, because apnea events can be surprisingly difficult to identify. In one study of 39 patients undergoing MAC, 10 (26%) developed 20 seconds of apnea, but none of these events was detected by the anesthesiologists in the study who were blinded to the capnography and thoracic impedance monitoring.[3] Consequently, all patients undergoing procedures in the Department of Radiology are monitored with equipment that has audible alarms that continually assesses the essential parameters of capnography, pulse oximetry, electrocardiography, and noninvasive blood pressure. For more complex procedures or critically ill patients, invasive arterial pressure monitoring sometimes is employed. All patients have intravenous access and receive supplemental oxygen. A defibrillator is immediately available for all patients as well as a "code cart" containing the required equipment and drugs for treating a compromised airway, cardiopulmonary arrest, anaphylaxis, or drug overdose. For procedures not staffed by an anesthesiologist, the nurse administering the sedation under the supervision of the interventional radiologist records the vital signs, drug dosing, drug administration times, and the sedation level of the patient in a contemporaneous fashion on a flow sheet that becomes part of the permanent medical record. (This contemporaneous recording is the responsibility of the anesthesiologist when MAC or GA is used.) Finally, all patients are transported to a dedicated recovery room after receiving procedural sedation. The recovery room is outfitted with continuous monitoring and support equipment and is staffed with appropriately trained personnel who observe the patients until they have regained their baseline level of consciousness and are no longer at risk for the cardiopulmonary complications of sedation.

Close collaboration between anesthesia and IR has led to other workplace safety and quality improvements. For example, it was previously standard practice to maintain very cool temperatures in the IR suites because cooler temperatures were thought to be "better" for the fluoroscopy equipment. The anesthesia staff was concerned that the low ambient temperatures unnecessarily increased the risk of hypothermia, particularly in elderly and sick patients. After checking with the manufacturers, it was determined that the temperature tolerance of the equipment was 68°F, so the thermostat was reset to this level. In addition, Bair Huggers (Arizant Healthcare Inc, Eden Prairie, Minnesota) now are used for all patients to maintain body temperature during procedures.

Conversely, the anesthesia staff has learned much about radiation safety and how to reduce personal radiation exposure. All anesthesia staff are required to wear lead, and floating into and out of the procedure room without proper lead protection is forbidden. The staff also has been advised to stay as far as possible from the radiation source during fluoroscopy and to leave the room or sit behind additional lead shielding during the acquisition of digital subtraction angiography.

QUALITY ASSURANCE SYSTEM

Other authors have stressed the importance of developing safety processes and quality assurance mechanisms to track events associated with procedural sedation performed outside the OR.[4,5] Within the authors' IR division, this process starts with interdisciplinary morning rounds, in which all the patients for the day are presented via an electronic scheduling program on a large liquid crystal display monitor in the reading room. The authors use the commercial system Hi-IQ (Conexsys, Ontario, Canada), an extremely powerful and versatile system designed for the modern IR practice. Hi-IQ integrates scheduling, electronic inventory management, case-flow monitoring, coding and billing, and quality management functions. The authors use Hi-IQ to store relevant data on the patient's history, to flag patients who need an anesthesia consultation, and to track all adverse events that occur, including those associated with procedural sedation. With this large database of information, the authors can review their caseload and complications efficiently in their monthly morbidity and mortality conference, thus facilitating root-cause analysis within IR and with the Department of Anesthesia. As mentioned previously, the hospital requires biennial recertification in ACLS and procedural sedation for all IR staff. In addition, a dedicated didactic session on procedural sedation is given annually by one of the board-certified anesthesiologists.

One remaining challenge is the development of a hospital-wide system for tracking events associated with procedural sedation and integrating the data so that they can be analyzed effectively and used to determine best-practice guidelines.

SERVICE THROUGHPUT

Certainly, the liability of the interventional radiologist or any other specialist performing minimally invasive procedures is reduced when an anesthesiologist assumes the responsibility for the procedural sedation. However, the authors have noticed that overall efficiency in terms of room turnover decreases significantly in cases requiring MAC or GA. While preprocedural assessment times have been reduced with the addition of the anesthesia nurse practitioners, inefficiencies remain when trying to coordinate teams from two different departments. This disadvantage could be mitigated by an interdepartmental electronic patient-tracking program for out-of-OR anesthesia cases similar to that already employed in the main OR, but the challenge of coordinating a centralized tracking system across several different departments is daunting.

SUMMARY

IR encompasses a broad and expanding array of image-guided, minimally invasive therapies that are essential to the practice of modern medicine. The growth and diversity of these non-OR procedures presents unique challenges and opportunities to anesthesiologists and interventional radiologists alike. Collaborative action has led to better patient care and quality management. Current trends indicate that non-OR anesthesia will become a significant component of patient care throughout the hospital and will become an even larger part of the overall anesthesia practice. It therefore is incumbent upon administrators and providers to ensure that all procedure rooms are safe for patients and allow for good, consistent anesthesia practice. This article has discussed why it will become increasingly necessary to expand the scope of pre-anesthesia evaluation. As the practice of non-OR anesthesia grows, it will be equally important to develop an effective mechanism of quality assurance that tracks patient outcomes across the hospital and, ultimately, across the health system. Finally, the practice of anesthesia in the IR suite and awareness of what the practice of anesthesiology offers must be incorporated into the curriculum of an anesthesia and IR training program, because it will be a major component of all integrated practice in the future.

REFERENCES

1. Gross JB, Bailey PL, Connis RT, et al. Practice guidelines for sedation and analgesia by non-anesthesiologists. Anesthesiology 2002;96(4):1004–17.
2. Bhananker SM, Posner KL, Cheney FW, et al. Injury and liability associated with monitored anesthesia care: a closed claims analysis. Anesthesiology 2006; 104(2):228–34.
3. Soto RG, Fu ES, Vila H Jr, et al. Capnography accurately detects apnea during monitored anesthesia care. Anesth Analg 2004;99(2):379–82.
4. Pino RM. The nature of anesthesia and procedural sedation outside of the operating room. Curr Opin Anaesthesiol 2007;20(4):347–51.
5. Kelly JS. Sedation by non-anesthesia personnel provokes safety concerns: anesthesiologists must balance JCAHO standards, politics, safety. Available at: http://www.apsf.org/resource_center/newsletter/2001/fall/07personnel.htm. Accessed May 25, 2008.

Fee for Service Payments: Affect on Patient Care, Operating Room Procedures and Anesthesia Services

Nancy M. Kane, DBA

KEYWORDS

• Medicare • Payment reform • Care fragmentation
• Bundling • Medical home

Medicare's traditional method of paying for units of service, be they hospital admissions, office visits, outpatient surgeries, or laboratory tests, evolved gradually from a payment system that originated in the 1930s, when private insurance for hospitalizations and physician services first emerged in this country. At that time, hospitals were just beginning to cure patients, emerging from their centuries-long primary function as almshouses that provided housing and minimal comforts to the sick poor. Desperate for capital resources, hospitals founded the first hospitalization insurance plans and designed their largely cost-based, open-ended payment systems to favor their own expansive growth. Physicians in the 1930s reluctantly joined private, largely physician-controlled insurance schemes to stave off compulsory public insurance. Fee-for-service was the payment system of choice for keeping insurers, with more restrictive or prescriptive forms of payment, out of the practice of medicine. Hospitalization and physician payment systems were designed to entice providers into accepting them, not to ensure that the right care was delivered at the right place and at the right time.

TOO MANY PAYMENT SILOS

The delivery system has come a long way since the 1930s, when the hospital was the physician's private workplace. As capital costs and technological advances have accelerated, hospitals, physicians, and other health care providers, willingly or not,

This article originally appeared in *Anesthesiology Clinics of North America*, Volume 27, Issue 1.
Harvard School of Public Health, 677 Huntington Avenue, Boston, MA 02115, USA
E-mail address: nkane@hsph.harvard.edu

Perioperative Nursing Clinics 4 (2009) 459–467
doi:10.1016/j.cpen.2009.09.011

have become increasingly interdependent, but current payment systems and medical culture do not reflect these changed relationships. Medicare's 18 separate payment systems for 16 different provider/supplier types, plus two types of private insurance plan (medical and drug) represent an elaborate scheme of "silos" that frequently pits the interest of one set of providers (eg, physicians) against the interests of another (eg, hospitals), leaving the patient in a daze, looking for an ombudsman.

PROLIFERATION AND FRAGMENTATION IN THE SITES OF TREATMENT

Changes in the sites of treatment have exacerbated fragmentation. Medicare expenditures for inpatient care have fallen from 50% of total traditional (non–managed care) spending in 1996 to only 34.5% in 2006.[1] In the same decade, Medicare spending for outpatient care rose from 4.5% to 8.3% of total traditional spending, and spending for "other fee-for-service settings" including hospice, outpatient laboratory, ambulatory surgical centers, and health clinics, grew from 11.2% to 15.5% of total traditional spending. For surgical procedures, the shift from hospital-based to free-standing ambulatory surgical centers (ASCs) has been dramatic: Medicare payments to ASCs doubled between 2000 and 2006, and the number of ASCs increased by more than 50% to 4707. Surgical care runs the risk of increased fragmentation with the proliferation of hospitals specializing in cardiac, orthopedic, and general surgeries. The number of such specialty hospitals grew from 46 to 89 between 2002 and 2004 and reached 130 in 2006 after the 2004–2005 moratorium on new specialty hospitals expired.[2] Even within hospitals, new "noninvasive, nonsurgical" approaches to disease via radiology and medical specialty clinics increase the likelihood of fragmentation by adding a whole new cadre of providers with whom the patient and the primary care-giver must interact, often without an infrastructure for doing so.

INCREASE IN THE NUMBER AND TYPES OF PHYSICIANS INVOLVED IN PROVIDING SERVICES

Even within the same payment silo (eg, physician services), the scope and number of providers involved in specialty treatment has increased the need for better care coordination. Within imaging services, for example, where growth in units of service per beneficiary has exploded in the last decade, radiologists now receive 43% of Medicare payments; the rest go to cardiologists (25%), surgical specialties (9%), independent diagnostic testing facilities (8%), internal medicine (6%), and other specialists (10%).

The average Medicare beneficiary sees five physicians a year. Nearly two thirds of Medicare beneficiaries with three or more common chronic conditions (eg, coronary artery disease, congestive heart failure, and diabetes) see 10 or more physicians in a year.[3] Yet fewer providers than ever are willing to spend the time, much of it unreimbursed, to coordinate care or communicate with the patient or other providers regarding the implications of the various tests and procedures provided.

Because of fragmentation, lack of coordination, and the fee-for-service incentives of Medicare payment, there is enormous variation in resource use and adherence to recognized quality standards and outcomes within severity-adjusted episodes. For instance, for similar severity-adjusted hypertensive patients, a high-cost cardiologist in Boston spends 1.74 times more on evaluation and management, 1.56 times more on imaging, and 1.39 times more on tests than the average Boston cardiologist. Similar variation occurs across metropolitan areas: in 2002, physicians in Boston treating Medicare patients for hypertension used 96% of the national average resource use per episode, whereas physicians in Houston and Miami used 120%, and those in Minneapolis used only 87% of the national average. Clinical quality measures show similar variation within and across cities, and they are not correlated highly with relative resource use.

OVERPAYMENT OF HIGHER-TECHNOLOGY CARE AT THE EXPENSE OF LOW-TECHNOLOGY CARE

Besides paying in silos that fail to align incentives across provider types (eg, hospital and physician) or within provider types (eg, radiologist and cardiologist, or proceduralist and anesthesiologist), Medicare also has an imperfect process for recognizing the impact of new technology on treatment cost and outcome. This deficiency affects care delivery in at least two ways. First, payment recognition for new technology involving physician services lags behind the appearance of that technology by several years, thereby slowing its adaptation. Second, payment adjustments for new technology that has been disseminated fully into practice, with the associated improvements in technique and scale, also are slow in coming, leaving in place incentives to overprovide newer technologies at the expense of equally or even more effective alternative treatments. The rapid migration of technically intensive procedures from operating rooms to non–operating room areas under the auspices of competing nonsurgical medical practitioners has strained the capabilities of payment systems to keep up with the proliferation of new service sites and types of practitioners.

The Resource-Based Relative Value System (RBRVS) assigns weights to physician service units (eg, office visit, diagnostic test, surgical procedure) based on the relative costliness of the inputs used to provide services: physician work, practice expense, and professional liability expenses. The relative weights for roughly 6700 distinct services in the Health care Common Procedural Coding System, the coding system for outpatient care under Medicare, are supposed to be updated at least every 5 years to reflect changes in medical practice, coding changes, new data, and the addition of new services. The minimum lead time for a new code can be several years; for instance, it is 18 months for new laboratory tests, but the service must be already "widely used" before the American Medical Association's Current Procedural Terminology Committee that supervises the coding system for insurance billing will consider it. Thus a test may be in the market for up to 2 years before it even can be submitted.[4]

On the other hand, Medicare has been slow to adjust relative weights downward once a new technology is well integrated into practice. Thus input costs generally are higher in the early years (when physician work may be more intensive or longer per treatment, patients involved may be more severely ill, and/or equipment or supply expenses may be higher because of lower volumes) than in later years when the service is well established and is being applied in higher volumes to less severely ill patients. The relative weights, however, are not lowered automatically to reflect the reduced input costs. A sign that Medicare has not done a good job of adjusting for the "experience curve" and impact of volume on new technology is the number of codes whose relative weights are reduced in 5-year reviews, relative to those that are increased. In 1996, for the first 5-year review following the 1992 introduction of the RBRVS system, the Resource Use Committee (RUC) of the American Medical Association, responsible for recommending relative weight changes to the Centers for Medicare and Medicaid Services, recommended increased weights for 296 codes, no change for 650 codes, and decreased weights for only 107 codes. At the second 5-year review in 2001, the RUC recommended increased weights for 469 codes, no change for 311 codes, and decreases for only 27. The Centers for Medicare and Medicaid Services accepted more than 90% of the RUC's recommendations.[5]

Because adjustments to relative weights are budget-neutral within the physician payment silo, increases in payment weights distribute the "fixed" resources more into the higher-weighted services while reducing the share of the pie paid to lower-weighted services. This system creates very strong incentives (overpayments) for physicians to provide more services with higher relative weights (services with newer technologies) and to avoid providing services with lower relative weights (services that do not use new technologies, such as evaluation and management or care coordination).

This "fee-for-service-on-steroids" phenomenon is responsible, at least in part, for fueling the enormous growth in the volume of high-technology services provided to Medicare beneficiaries in recent years. Between 2000 and 2005, the cumulative volume of physician services per beneficiary increased 30%, with the greatest increases in imaging (61%) and tests (46%). These volume increases have fueled large, politically unpopular increases in Medicare Part B premiums and are largely responsible for the negative updates in the physician fee schedule that are required by current law. At the same time, evaluation and management services, which include vital but underprovided services such as care coordination and patient education, had the lowest per-beneficiary rate of increase over the 5-year period—less than 20%.

Relatively poor payment for coordination and other primary care services has contributed to a severe shortage of United States medical school graduates willing to enter primary care residencies.[6] Although foreign medical graduates have been willing to fill the gap in recent years, the difference in income between primary and specialty practice is growing, and this difference will aggravate a predicted shortage of primary care physicians just as the baby-boomers reach Medicare age with a host of chronic care needs.[7]

IMPROVING INTEGRATION OF CARE ACROSS AND WITHIN PAYMENT SYSTEMS: POTENTIAL REFORMS
The Problem of the Sustainable Growth Rate Formula Is Absorbing Policy Attention with no Remedy in Sight

Much of the recent policy debate about physician payment involves eliminating the Sustainable Growth Rate (SGR) constraint on physician fees. The SGR was imposed by Congress in the Balanced Budget Act of 1997, limiting growth in Medicare physician expenditures per beneficiary to inflation plus the per capita growth in gross domestic product using 1996 as the base year. Total physician expenditures have exceeded this limit since 2001, thereby mandating across-the-board cuts in physician fees since 2002. As of 2008, however, Congress has overridden its own mandate in all but one of the last 7 years; each delay in implementing the law creates an ever-deeper deficit to be recovered out of future years' physician expenditures. The cumulative SGR deficit has grown so large (more than $60 billion as of 2007) that at least 9 years of 5% fee cuts each year would be needed to comply with the law. Trustees of the Medicare Trust Fund have called this projected series of negative updates "unrealistically low," but Congress has not yet come up with an alternative, budget-neutral way to address the problem. Meanwhile, the fees not cut do not keep up with inflation and encourage even greater volume growth, although the greater volume per beneficiary does not seem to be related to better outcomes or better patient satisfaction with care.[8] Finally, although the fee-for-service system strongly encourages more volume, which is not needed, it does not reward care coordination or high-quality care, which is urgently needed.

It Is Time to Focus on Alternatives to Fee-for-Service in Provider Silos

Although there is some truth in the popular joke that the most expensive piece of technology in a hospital is the physician's pen, the reality is that other parties are encouraged by their payment systems to provide a greater volume of service without regard to quality of care, overall cost, or health care maintenance. Hospitals have strong incentives to admit patients and to increase the care they provide in the less constrained outpatient setting, as well as to discharge patients early. Postacute providers have strong incentives keep patients Medicare-eligible even if that means re-admitting them to acute hospitals for the requisite 3-day stay for conditions that otherwise might have been treated more effectively in a community-based or long-term care setting. Equipment and pharmaceutical suppliers are paid only if their products are used, so they engage in direct-to-consumer advertising and marketing campaigns directed at physicians. One of the biggest problems in traditional Medicare is that no one is held accountable for the quality or cost of the entire package of services delivered to a beneficiary during an episode of illness or a year of chronic disease. Worse still, no one is held responsible for keeping Medicare beneficiaries healthy.

The Medicare Payment Advisory Commission (MedPAC) has recommended to Congress a number of reforms that would begin to address provider accountability for services outside the provider's service and/or payment silo. Two of these reforms are described here, because they reflect the most recent discussions and recommendations to Congress in the spring of 2008. A third concept described here is not yet at the recommendation stage but is complementary to the other two. The three would represent significant change in the way delivery systems are structured and operated. Their potential impact, if enacted, could be much more far reaching than the 1983 payment reform that replaced retrospective cost-based reimbursement with prospective diagnosis-related group payments for inpatient care. That reform contributed to a 20-year decline in inpatient days (and related inpatient capacity), as well as to an explosion in the development and use of outpatient and postacute providers. Given the potential impact of these possible reforms, it is likely that their implementation, if passed, would take several years. Even with a phased-in implementation, however, it is likely that some institutions will adapt and thrive, and others will not.

Bundling Parts A and B for High-Cost, High-Volume Inpatient Admissions

MedPAC's April 2008 recommendation to Congress, unanimously adopted, reads as follows:[9]

> To encourage providers to collaborate and better coordinate care, the Congress should direct the Secretary (of HHS) to reduce payments to hospitals with relatively high readmission rates for select conditions and also allow shared accountability between physicians and hospitals. The Congress should also direct the Secretary to report within two years on the feasibility of broader approaches such as virtual bundling for encouraging efficiency across hospitalization episodes. The Congress should require the Secretary to create a voluntary pilot program to test the feasibility of actual bundled payments for services around hospitalization episodes for select conditions. The pilot must have clear and explicit thresholds for determining if it can be expanded into the full Medicare program, or discontinued entirely.

Under bundled payment, Medicare would pay a single entity (one in which all providers involved were represented) an amount that would cover the expected costs of providing all services for the hospitalization and related postacute period. This proposal could be implemented on a pilot/voluntary basis for organizations with an infrastructure already capable of receiving and allocating bundled payments. For those lacking such an infrastructure, a phased approach could include, first, a confidential information-only strategy and eventually incorporate mandatory bonuses and penalties within a fee-for-service withhold system ("virtual" bundling).

Bundled payment might begin by focusing primarily on holding hospitals, physicians, and postacute providers responsible for 30-day readmission rates, which vary from 13% to 24% depending on the state.[10] This plan would encourage hospitals to work with physicians and postacute providers to re-engineer the care process, addressing mortality, morbidity, readmission rates, and costs throughout the patient's hospitalization and recovery experience. A bundled payment system would encourage providers to do a better job of coordinating and communicating through hand-offs of patients through the process of care and across the traditional payment silos. Focusing on inpatient admissions as the trigger for bundling also targets the most costly Medicare beneficiaries; the most costly 20% of Medicare beneficiaries average 1.7 admissions per year.

Medical Homes

In the same April 2008 meeting, MedPAC Commissioners also unanimously supported the following recommendations to Congress:[10]

> Congress should initiate a medical home pilot project in Medicare. Eligible medical homes must meet stringent criteria, including at least the following: Furnish primary care, including coordinating appropriate preventive, maintenance and acute health services; use health information technology for active clinical decision support; conduct care management; maintain 24-hour patient communication and rapid access; keep up to-date records of patient's advanced directives; have a formal quality improvement program; maintain a written understanding with beneficiary designating the provider as a medical home.
>
> Medicare should provide medical homes with timely data on patient use. The pilot should require a physician pay-for-performance program. Finally, the pilot must have clear and explicit thresholds for determining if it can be expanded into the full Medicare program, or discontinued entirely.

Under a medical home arrangement, the designated provider would be paid a monthly capitation for providing comprehensive, continuous care and acting as a resource for helping patients and families navigate through the health system to select optimal treatments and providers. The provider would continue to be paid fee-for-service for providing Part B services, subject to a pay-for-performance component reflecting the provider's clinical quality and efficient use of resources. Specialists could qualify as a medical home when they sign up to manage specific chronic diseases of their patients, such as a cardiologist managing patients who have congestive heart failure, or endocrinologists managing the care of diabetics. The provider's efficient and effective use of resources ultimately would affect participation and payment levels in the medical home program.

Eligibility might be limited at first to beneficiaries who have at least two chronic conditions, and enrollment in a medical home would be voluntary. Beneficiaries still would be free to see specialists without a referral from the medical home, although they might have an obligation to inform the medical home of their use of a non–medical home provider. There would be no beneficiary cost sharing for medical home fees.

Medical homes would begin to address the fact that beneficiaries with chronic conditions do not receive recommended care and are sometimes hospitalized for events that could have been prevented with better primary care. Researchers have found that adult patients who have chronic conditions receive recommended care only 56% of the time.[11] Avoidable Medicare hospitalizations related to congestive heart failure, chronic obstructive pulmonary disease, hypertension, and three forms of complications for uncontrolled diabetes are among the top 12 reasons for Medicare hospitalizations.[12] One study found that 38% of patients without chronic disease experienced medical mistakes, that is, medication and laboratory errors caused by lack of coordination across care settings. Even more patients (48%) reported similar mistakes when four or more doctors were involved in their care.[13] Although medical homes will not solve all the problems caused by fragmentation, fee-for-service silos, and lack of incentives for physicians to work collaboratively to improve patient care, they at least are headed in the right direction.

Accountable Care Organizations

Although MedPAC made no recommendations to Congress regarding accountable care organizations (ACOs), the concept was discussed extensively as a means of controlling excessive volume growth and addressing the uneven quality of care provided to all Medicare beneficiaries, not just those who have chronic or acute conditions. An ACO would be a group of physicians, possibly including a hospital, that is responsible for quality and overall Medicare spending for their patients over the course of a year. It could involve fee-for-service payment with withholds, penalties, and bonuses, or could move into more bundled payment designs if an infrastructure is created to allocate payments across provider types. ACOs would be responsible for all patients within a geographic area who agree to participate, thus expanding the concept of bundling beyond medical homes and bundled hospitalization care to include well-care, prevention, and health maintenance. They could be voluntary groups of physicians who choose to work together or who are within the same hospital's primary service area, or they could be already established multispecialty group practices.

Many philosophical and practical issues regarding the implementation of ACOs remain to be worked out, ranging from whether they should be voluntary (in which case there could be selection bias) or mandatory (which would generate high resistance in many unstructured markets), whether they should include hospitals, and whether nonparticipating physicians would continue to have their fee updates subject to the SGR. The direction of the policy discussion clearly is to encourage broader provider accountability across the payment silos for patient cost, quality, and outcomes.

SUMMARY

The rising tide of uninsured and underinsured Americans is a sign that the health care financing system is broken. Many policymakers, providers, and beneficiaries, however, believe that the health care delivery system is broken, too. To the extent that the present payment systems contribute to the high cost, poor quality, and lack of accountability that characterizes today's health care delivery system, there is hope that reforms are within reach. Medicare, as the largest payer in the country, can lead the way, as it did with diagnosis-related groups and RBRVUs, to change fundamentally the dynamics of health delivery in the United States. Already private insurers are experimenting with care coordination, provider accountability, and pay-for-performance concepts on a smaller scale. Some are hampered in their efforts to distinguish high-cost and poor-quality providers effectively because of the relatively small numbers of patients per provider. Medicare could increase substantially the validity and credibility of the tools of provider accountability by combining its beneficiary population data and its technical expertise with those of private-sector insurers. The technical ability to identify episodes of acute and chronic illness and to link providers to clinical measures of care and outcomes is improving every day, making payment reforms linked to meaningful measures of performance increasingly possible.

The implications for providers are that payment incentives of the future are likely to favor care coordination; information systems; integration/collaboration across primary, inpatient, and postacute sectors; performance measurement; and re-engineered processes of care. Obviously a big challenge is timing; the old payment incentives to provide ever-higher volumes of care continue, and they continue to punish those who do "the right thing." Physicians seeking to maximize volume and intensity of services at the expense of appropriate, high-quality patient care will resist efforts to hold them accountable for outcomes such as readmissions and unexpected complications. Hospitals that fail to see the need to build a collaborative, interdisciplinary infrastructure that improves patient care across the silos will struggle along the same path that led to the demise of their predecessors who were unable to manage their lengths of stay in the 1980s. Forward-looking hospital systems already are experimenting with integrated physician–hospital care packages in the private sector (eg, Geisinger Health System's extended episode warranty on coronary bypass surgery)[14] and in Medicare Demonstration projects (eg, the Acute Care Episode demonstration project and the Hospital Gainsharing Project).[15] Achieving fundamental reform of the health care system to improve patient outcomes will take decades of effort and a major shift in financial, medical, and political behaviors that have built up since the beginning of health insurance in the United States. In retrospect, managing length of stay was a piece of cake!

REFERENCES

1. Medicare Payment Advisory Commission. Data Book. Washington, DC: Medicare Payment Advisory Commission; 2007. p. 9, 116, 118, 104. Available at: http://www.medpac.gov.
2. Medicare Payment Advisory Commission. Report to Congress specialty hospitals revisited. Washington, DC: Medicare Payment Advisory Commission; 2006. p. 4.
3. Medicare Payment Advisory Commission. Report to the Congress, increasing the value of medicare. Washington, DC: Medicare Payment Advisory Commission; 2006. p. 36, 107, 108.
4. Quinn B. Crossing the three chasms: complex molecular testing and Medicare regulations. Foley Hoag LLP, Boston.
5. Medicare Payment Advisory Commission. Report to the congress medicare payment policy. Washington, DC: Medicare Payment Advisory Commission; 2006. p. 142.
6. Bodenheimer. Primary care—will it survive? N Engl J Med 2006;355(9):861–4.
7. Tu HT, O'Malley AS. Exodus of male physicians from primary care drives shift to specialty practice: tracking report no. 17. Center for Studying Health System Change. Available at: http://www.hschange.org/CONTENT/934/. Accessed November 29, 2008.
8. Fisher E. The implications of regional variations in medicare spending. Part 2: health outcomes and satisfaction with care. Ann Intern Med 2003;138(4):273–87.
9. Meeting of the Medicare Payment Advisory Commission [transcript]. Washington, DC, April 9, 2008. p. 300–1.
10. Cantor JC, Belloff D, Schoen C, et al. "Aiming higher" results from a state scorecard on health system performance, commonwealth fund. Available at: http://www.com

monwealthfund.org/publications/publications_show.htm?doc_id=494551. 2007. Accessed June 10, 2008.

11. McGlynn EA, Asch SM, Adams J, et al. The quality of health care delivered to adults in the United States. N Engl J Med 2003;348(26):2635–45.

12. Rich MW, Beckham V, Wittenberg C, et al. A multidisciplinary intervention to prevent the reasmission of elderly patients with congestive heart failure. N Engl J Med 1995;333(18):1190–5.

13. Schoen C, Osborn R, Huynh PT, et al. Taking the pulse of health care systems: experiences of patients with health problems in six countries. Health affairs web exclusive (not 3). Available at: http://www.healthaffairs.org. Accessed June 16, 2008.

14. Available at: http://www.nytimes.com/2007/05/17/business/17quality.html. Accessed August 12, 2008.

15. Available at: http://www.cms.hhs.gov/demoprojectsevalrpts/md/list.asp?listpage=2. Accessed August 12, 2008.

Index

Note: Page numbers of article titles are in **bold face** type.

A

Abdominal cancer pain, celiac plexus neurolysis for, 339–340
Accountable care organizations, 465
Acetaminophen, 377, 379, 382, 386
Adenosine receptor activation, 394
Allodynia, clinical examination in, 329
Alpha-adrenoreceptor antagonists, topical, 396
Amethocaine, topical, 393
Amitriptyline, topical, 394–395
Amputation, phantom phenomena in, motor cortex stimulation for, 342–343
Analgesia
    nonopioid, **377–389**
    SAFE score for, 371–373
    spinal, 337–339
    topical, **391–403**
    translational, 367–372
Anesthesia
    for gastrointestinal endoscopy, **421–435, 437–450**
    for interventional radiology, **451–458**
    for non-hospital settings, monitoring in, **405–420**
        blood pressure measurement, 410–411
        capnography, 407–410
        controversies in, 413–415
        electrocardiography, 411
        electroencephalography, 411
        in angiography, 413
        in computed tomography room, 412
        in electroconvulsive therapy, 412
        in endoscopy suite, 412–413
        in magnetic resonance imaging suite, 412
        pulse oximetry, 406–407
        recommendations for, 415–416
        temperature, 411
    payment for, **459–467**
Angiography, 413, 453
Antidepressants, tricyclic, topical application of, 394–396
Anti-inflammatory action, of nonopioid analgesics, 379
Antipyretic action, of nonopioid analgesics, 379
Appendectomy, with natural orifice transluminal endoscopic surgery, 442–443
Aspirin, 378–379, 381–382
Attentional training, for pain management, 320

Perioperative Nursing Clinics 4 (2009) 469–477
doi:10.1016/S1556-7931(09)00084-9
1556-7931/09/$ – see front matter © 2009 Elsevier Inc. All rights reserved.
periopnursing.theclinics.com

United States Postal Service

Statement of Ownership, Management, and Circulation
(All Periodicals Publications Except Requestor Publications)

1. Publication Title	2. Publication Number	3. Filing Date
Perioperative Nursing Clinics	0 2 4 - 5 3 3 5	9/15/09

4. Issue Frequency	5. Number of Issues Published Annually	6. Annual Subscription Price
Mar, Jun, Sep, Dec	4	$116.00

7. Complete Mailing Address of Known Office of Publication (Not printer) (Street, city, county, state, and ZIP+4®)

Elsevier Inc.
360 Park Avenue South
New York, NY 10010-1710

Contact Person: Stephen Bushing
Telephone (Include area code): 215-239-3688

8. Complete Mailing Address of Headquarters or General Business Office of Publisher (Not printer)

Elsevier Inc., 360 Park Avenue South, New York, NY 10010-1710

9. Full Names and Complete Mailing Addresses of Publisher, Editor, and Managing Editor (Do not leave blank)

Publisher (Name and complete mailing address)

John Schrefer, Elsevier, Inc., 1600 John F. Kennedy Blvd. Suite 1800, Philadelphia, PA 19103-2899

Editor (Name and complete mailing address)

Katie Hartner, Elsevier, Inc., 1600 John F. Kennedy Blvd. Suite 1800, Philadelphia, PA 19103-2899

Managing Editor (Name and complete mailing address)

Catherine Bewick, Elsevier, Inc., 1600 John F. Kennedy Blvd. Suite 1800, Philadelphia, PA 19103-2899

10. Owner (Do not leave blank. If the publication is owned by a corporation, give the name and address of the corporation immediately followed by the names and addresses of all stockholders owning or holding 1 percent or more of the total amount of stock. If not owned by a corporation, give the names and addresses of the individual owners. If owned by a partnership or other unincorporated firm, give its name and address as well as those of each individual owner. If the publication is published by a nonprofit organization, give its name and address.)

Full Name	Complete Mailing Address
Wholly owned subsidiary of	4520 East-West Highway
Reed/Elsevier, US holdings	Bethesda, MD 20814

11. Known Bondholders, Mortgagees, and Other Security Holders Owning or Holding 1 Percent or More of Total Amount of Bonds, Mortgages, or Other Securities. If none, check box ☐ None

Full Name	Complete Mailing Address
N/A	

12. Tax Status (For completion by nonprofit organizations authorized to mail at nonprofit rates) (Check one)
The purpose, function, and nonprofit status of this organization and the exempt status for federal income tax purposes:
☐ Has Not Changed During Preceding 12 Months
☐ Has Changed During Preceding 12 Months (Publisher must submit explanation of change with this statement)

PS Form 3526, September 2007 (Page 1 of 3 (Instructions Page 3)) PSN 7530-01-000-9931 PRIVACY NOTICE: See our Privacy policy in www.usps.com

---

13. Publication Title	14. Issue Date for Circulation Data Below
Perioperative Nursing Clinics	September 2009

15. Extent and Nature of Circulation		Average No. Copies Each Issue During Preceding 12 Months	No. Copies of Single Issue Published Nearest to Filing Date
a. Total Number of Copies (Net press run)		688	650
b. Paid Circulation (By Mail and Outside the Mail)	(1) Mailed Outside-County Paid Subscriptions Stated on PS Form 3541. (Include paid distribution above nominal rate, advertiser's proof copies, and exchange copies)	256	194
	(2) Mailed In-County Paid Subscriptions Stated on PS Form 3541 (Include paid distribution above nominal rate, advertiser's proof copies, and exchange copies)		
	(3) Paid Distribution Outside the Mails Including Sales Through Dealers and Carriers, Street Vendors, Counter Sales, and Other Paid Distribution Outside USPS®	7	6
	(4) Paid Distribution by Other Classes Mailed Through the USPS (e.g. First-Class Mail®)		
c. Total Paid Distribution (Sum of 15b (1), (2), (3), and (4))	▶	263	200
d. Free or Nominal Rate Distribution (By Mail and Outside the Mail)	(1) Free or Nominal Rate Outside-County Copies Included on PS Form 3541	54	57
	(2) Free or Nominal Rate In-County Copies Included on PS Form 3541		
	(3) Free or Nominal Rate Copies Mailed at Other Classes Through the USPS (e.g. First-Class Mail)		
	(4) Free or Nominal Rate Distribution Outside the Mail (Carriers or other means)		
e. Total Free or Nominal Rate Distribution (Sum of 15d (1), (2), (3) and (4))	▶	54	57
f. Total Distribution (Sum of 15c and 15e)	▶	317	257
g. Copies not Distributed (See instructions to publishers #4 (page #3))	▶	371	393
h. Total (Sum of 15f and g)	▶	688	650
i. Percent Paid (15c divided by 15f times 100)		82.97%	77.82%

16. Publication of Statement of Ownership
☐ If the publication is a general publication, publication of this statement is required. Will be printed in the December 2009 issue of this publication. ☐ Publication not required

17. Signature and Title of Editor, Publisher, Business Manager, or Owner

Stephen R. Bushing

Stephen R. Bushing – Subscription Services Coordinator

Date: September 15, 2009

I certify that all information furnished on this form is true and complete. I understand that anyone who furnishes false or misleading information on this form or who omits material or information requested on the form may be subject to criminal sanctions (including fines and imprisonment) and/or civil sanctions (including civil penalties).

PS Form 3526, September 2007 (Page 2 of 3)

Moving?

Make sure your subscription moves with you!

To notify us of your new address, find your **Clinics Account Number** (located on your mailing label above your name), and contact customer service at:

Email: journalscustomerservice-usa@elsevier.com

800-654-2452 (subscribers in the U.S. & Canada)
314-447-8871 (subscribers outside of the U.S. & Canada)

Fax number: 314-447-8029

Elsevier Health Sciences Division
Subscription Customer Service
3251 Riverport Lane
Maryland Heights, MO 63043

*To ensure uninterrupted delivery of your subscription, please notify us at least 4 weeks in advance of move.

Printed and bound by CPI Group (UK) Ltd, Croydon, CR0 4YY

03/10/2024

01040462-0015